SAD DRESSING GOWN

It was hung up on the back of the door

Very threadbare, very worn,

Ragged and torn

Just shades of reds and blues

Coming through

So sad to see it hanging there,

Many years have passed

But still it is worn

Its owner has no other, this one must last

Every night without fail

This dressing gown must prevail

There is no money to replace it

So threads so worn,

Its rags unable to keep poor John warm

But, still the dressing gown

Without its look

Returns each night upon its hook.

Beauty's Shelf Life

Standing there so pretty, men look twice, maybe three times, but always that look that nod, that smile, but always a stare. She knows it, loves it, hunger's for it, her power, her enchantment capturing that knowing look, that stare.

Over time, it still happens, that look, but from a different generation now, not the young men, but older ones, thirties, forties, she still longs for that look from them. Gone out with one or two, still looking for that Mr Right, will he be there? She searches, endless conversations, endless chats, dinners, pubs, cinemas, nightclubs, but nothing, he is not there.

She moves on in time, the pubs, clubs, bars are less, still the look, the stare, and still she is aware, but it's an even older generation, her hair tied back, long still, but greyer, she does not bother much, what's the point, no one out there, just an emptiness a void, nothing, he does not exist, or maybe he did at some point, but she was too young, did not understand had no idea, this word 'compromise', that nothing is perfect, it is a myth, all habits come too.

Still she walks, still her looks are there, not so powerful anymore, she doesn't care, he isn't there, and she has given up. The stares less frequent, and when they come, she is surprised, her hair is greyer, her eyes are sadder, her face is lined, her walk is stooped, but now and again that look is given, her power going, fading with time.

She walks alone, slowly now, her time has gone, her chance, the window of opportunity shut, tightly closed, she waits now, waiting for what? Did she miss out? Was there something out there, her Mr Right, or is this only a distance hope spun out as a joke, only emptiness?

She walks not far now, just enough a few steps, her hair is tied back, just a few strands fall free, her hands hold onto a stick, there are no stares, no looks. She is now passed her sell by date, disposed of in the bin, no hope, her time has gone by.

'Hello there,' a voice calls to her from the dark, a withered, weather, beaten old man appears, a stick much larger than her own, no hair, no teeth, eyes blurred, 'you have a beautiful face. Would you take a walk with me, share a cup of tea, a biscuit, pass some time,' he asked.

Is this my Mr Right? A hand is held out, a withered, lined, vein hand, she reaches for it. She misses, she falls. Her stick thrown to the side lay on the grassy verge, her frail crumbled body lies on its side.

'Are you alright?' he asks.

She looks up with wide open eyes, and sees his face, his smile. 'Yes, thank you, I am fine,' she says, lying still on the cold, hard ground.

The voice is silent, the hard ground turns soft and warm, soft mellow music plays on. There is nothing now, it's gone, quietness, a dark shadow, no light, no hope, just gone, sleep comes, her eyes are closed, one last thought before the door is shut, 'what was it all for, this beauty in life, nothing lasts it's only a game.'

John's workplace No Shame

The brand new top of the range Volvo over thirty thousand pounds worth of car, was parked outside the workshop, five minutes later another one appeared, then another until there were four of them, all lined up outside the workshop, these gleaming white cars, the smell of leather wafted through the cold workshop towards John's nose.

John who was hurdled up over his work bench, stripping down televisions with his cold hands, with each breath a ringlet of steam oozed out into the cold air, he looked out across the car park, and watched them walking around their cars, playing with their remote controls, the side mirrors going back and forwards, the electronic lights switching off and on. John stood up and reached for his coat, he pulled it around him, and sat back on the hard bench, peering at a tiny micro chip, he fiddled around but his fingers too cold to hold the small tool, he placed it back on the bench and blew hard on his fingers willing them to warm up.

They came back into the shop, 'morning,' one shouts to John at the back of the workshop, 'could I have a word with you if you have a minute?' said, one of the directors, John's boss. John was only to please to get up and go into the warm heated office, his fingers tingled as the sensation returned to his blue numb finger tips, the fan heater blew hot air around the small room.

'It's about your bonus this year, well I am sorry to say that we haven't made enough money this year to pay it out to you. You see it's like this John, well, times are hard I am afraid,' the Director said, as he sat back in his two hundred and thirty pound massage office chair, his heavy bulk spreading out like a walrus just lumbered up from the sea.

John looked down at his fingers as he they came to life with the warmth, and then at the keys placed casually on the desk, the shiny logo off Volvo seemed to taunt him, tease him. 'And, about your pay rise, well that is on hold as well,' said the fat balding director, 'no money in the pot, well you know how it is, chocolate biscuit?'

Before John's lifeless fingers could make a grab at the offered chocolate biscuit, the tin was snatched back. The biscuit was consumed within seconds every chocolaty finger licked clean.

The keys with the shining Volvo tab seemed to come to life, they lifted off the table and danced around in front of John, 'we appreciate all the long hours you have put into this company, and the hard work you have done,' the director's voice droned on and on, 'and we were sorry to hear about your back, but we feel it wasn't the large LCD television that you installed on your own, that caused the injury, no we think it was some ongoing problem you had before you came here.'

The shinning keys moved in front of John's eyes, they jingled and danced, 'and about the Christmas party, well that is off as well.' John pulled his coat around him, knowing that soon he would leave the director's heated office, and return to his own damp cold bench with the icy wind howling around the open workshop door.

'How is your car?' the director asked, 'I hear you have been late for work a couple of mornings.'

John's gaze returned to the fat podgy director's face. He looked at the balding man in front of him, the gold rings on his sausage fingers, the expensive gold watched, and then at the photos on the wall behind him, a recent one of golfing holiday in America.

'My car is off the road,' said John, 'I have had to use my bike, but I had a puncture in the tyre this morning, so I walked to work.' The director hadn't heard John, he was shuffling some invoices with cheques stapled to them, payment for work that John had done.

John thought about his battered old car, if it wasn't for the tape and the plaster, it would fall apart; the seats were thread bare, coils of rusty springs showing through, rust upon rust, and two engines in two years, with each one falling apart.

'Please make sure you are here on time. Perhaps you could leave earlier in the morning to get here on time then,' the director suggested, picking up a cheque and examining it in great detail, then placed it back down on the desk.

'Two thousand pounds for a television and installation that I did, maybe when I damaged my back,' John thought to himself.

'Get up early,' John mulled these words over in his head, thinking to himself, 'well I get up at two thirty now to do my Sainsbury's job, cleaning the floors for three hours, then I come here and do a full day's work, and get home have my tea, let me see,' John reflected over his life in his head, 'yes for tea, my cheese sandwich, on basic Tesco bread, with plastic cheese. If I get up any earlier I might as well not go to bed,' John thought, he looked back down at the desk the silver shiny brand new Volvo keys looked back at him, but they were moving again, coming closer towards him,.

He heard the director's voice, 'so you will make sure you are on time then John, can't have you late you know, you must get yourself sorted out. There is no room for laziness here. Well I must go now and get ready, going away, golf meeting, plane to catch. The states Florida, warm this time of year.'

The keys jumped into John's hand, he felt the cold hard metal press into his palms. The keys had strength. They came to a sharp point, the director sat back, 'well that is all John, what are you waiting for?'

The keys appeared to be moving again, taking John's hand with it, he couldn't control them. They had a mind of their own. They were pulling his hand, his arm, his body, he couldn't stop them, they were stronger than him, 'oh my God, they have stabbed the director in the left eye. 'Fuck you,' the keys shouted.

No Birthday Card from my Daughter

Hope was there, as the letter box clicked, two brown envelopes nothing more, no birthday card today. Just one single card stood on the mantel piece, alone, there should have been four. Those days, of smiles and laughter, as sticky handmade cards, were placed on the bed covers long gone. Instead a shop bought card with shop bought words, read Happy Birthday, not real, not meant, just words, exchanged for money.

The three missing cards scream 'we forgot' a hole where now only emptiness stands. We shouldn't have cards, no birthday wishes, it's just a passing of a year, is it worth a celebration, or should we pass on the good years?

A missing card shouts a thousand words; just best it was left without the cheers, then no guilt, no sadness, nothing missing, just another passing day. But, each one of us is guilty of that need to purchase a birthday card a sign of thinking of your day. What day? Another day where human misery exists, laden high with guilt that stuck on a planet, full of sorrow, no hope for tomorrow, only pain, anguish we have caused, by simple forgetting or choosing to ignore, another human being, not perfect, but with flaws.

This is human nature, to feel guilt, did she forget? Or not worth a thought, a shop bought thought, not from the heart, the little white cards sold for a few pence.

A passing of a birthday, without a card, shouts out loud, that 'you're not worth it; I didn't buy a card for you, because the bottom line is I'm not you. You maybe my mother, my mum, but not buying that card shows to you how glum I am that my mother is not the one I want. I am telling you that I was switch at birth. Wrong baby, wrong child, how can you be my mum?'

Families are hard work, we try our best, but what's it for? An empty mantel piece that's all, a card that's missing shouts to you, you may be my mother, but I don't want you.

The pain this creates, when not sending that card, is such a powerful statement, it can turn to hate. But, I know deep down, she is sore, with me, her mother, the one I bore, no longer likes this person I am, wants to exchange me for a better one.

The birthday's now gone; another day moved on, a single card removed, taken down from the mantel piece. What next? What hope does the future have, when the arguments are mistaken for a hate, when really deep down, the love a mother has for her child, is unstoppable, like a burst dam, never faltering always there, birthday cards not bought, will not stop a mother's love.

There's hope for the next time, when a card will flutter though a letter box, lands on the mat, a show of how I remember you on this day, for a few pence I pay to show my mum how I love her, she makes mistakes, but that's ok, she's after all only human. No saint, no higher order, just a mother who loves her daughter.

Photo

Every Sunday morning, at nine o'clock, he leaves the small cottage for his walk. This morning, was no different, he places his mug on the table, rose, walks into the hall and takes his coat a large brown coat off the peg, and fastens it tight. His thick black boots were already on his feet, so all that was left was the camera on the kitchen table. This he picks up the last item, always in that order every Sunday.

The wind was quite blustery, fresh off the sea, an easterly wind, the one with a bit of a bite to it. The sun was late rising over the distant marshlands, a small band of grey thick cloud partially covers the watery sun, and so only the orange tips peek through like long tentacles, snaking out each one omitting a deep orange glow.

The long marshy grasses were soaked from the heavy rain fall last evening, but he walks with firm strides a man with a purpose. I follow behind him; I always do unable to keep up with his long legs. I shout across, 'wait for me,' but the wind whips my words away, gone across the rugged recently ploughed fields.

He climbs up the dyke and stands proudly on the top, surveying the scene around him; a flock of sea gulls sit on the wet marsh lands, the recent high tide only just receding, their eager beaks pecking away at the delights left by the fast flowing sea waters. 'You could have waited,' I call across to him; he turns around and smiles, then takes his camera and points it towards me. I smile back, he was always photographing, either birds, skies, or just the flat marsh lands.

He takes a few more shots, while I sit on a wooden log, part of a fence torn up by the weather, now discarded on the edge of the grassy dyke. I take time to look around, the sun finally manages to throw away the grey clouds, edge its way higher into the sky, but in late November it never really manages to throw any warmth, the wind's bite now penetrating my thin cotton jacket. 'Why didn't I put my thick coat on?' I ask myself, as I pull the thin material around my neck, 'and this tee-shirt underneath is ridiculous this time of the year. What was I thinking coming out here dressed like this?'

He tucks his camera away in its heavy black case, swung it over his neck and walks back across the fields. 'This is my favourite place to,' I call over to him, but once again the wind rips my words away. 'I love this spot, where the river meets the sea, and if you stand on this sand bank here, look right here,' I call over towards him, 'you can just make out the tip of Spurn Point in Yorkshire.'

He is sitting on a bench. I do not remember the bench that is new. I come closer; a recent bench not at all weather worn. There is a name engraved on the back of the seat, but without my glasses it is hopeless, I can't read the name and the dates, but hang on a minute that date twenty third of July, I know that date funny it is the same date as my birthday.

He is walking on now. Walking back towards the cottage, how I love that cottage so warm and inviting on blustery days like today. I catch up with him; my small footsteps follow in his large imprints.

I stand and look over his shoulder, he is staring at the photograph in his hand the one he took of me earlier.

'Oh my god,' I think to myself, as I look at it. I lean over to have another look, 'why have I so many strange lines around my face?' I ask him, 'this is not like you to take a bad photograph.' I stand back and look up at the wall above his desk. There hanging is a photograph taken not so long ago of me standing in the same spot that he took of me this morning, but the photograph on the wall is different.

In that photo I am smiling into his camera, my brown eyes shine down, my long brown hair blowing in the wind, he caught me as I stood looking across the marshes. That same spot as the one he took of me this morning, the one he now has in his hand. My face is lined, but these are strange lines, as though half my face is missing, between those lines, a yellow faded line. 'These are not my eyes,' I say, as I look down at the photograph once more. 'I don't have black eyes. What have you done?' I ask him again, my voice sounds a higher pitch than normal.

He turns around; he is looking at me, not wait through me. He holds the photograph between his fingers; he walks across to the fire. 'What are you doing?' I call across to him, as he tosses it into the flames. He sits and watches as the hungry logs devour the photo, until the last crinkled piece withers and dies. I sit down next to him, and watch the photo as it turns to dust. A gust of wind blows the door wide open, I feel myself being pulled towards it. Higher and higher I go.

Chased

It was one of those very wet days not with rain, but with low cloud, a thick heavy mist that hung low over the valley, like a carpet concealing a beautiful mosaic floor. The van pulled off the main road and onto a dirt track leading into a wooded area. The ground was sodden from the evening's heavy downpour; the warm air lifted the moisture to create a stubborn mist.

The back wheels get stuck for a few minutes, then with heavy revving they freed themselves, giving a violent jolt to the cargo at the back, a sickening thud indicated a few bashed bodies, but nothing more. Two more black four by fours followed the van up the track. These heavy vehicles were able to negotiate the waterlogged potholes.

My stomach was tense with anticipation and excitement; it always was on such occasions, the only thing spoiling it this morning was the weather. A clearing came into view where trees once stood tall and proud, lay broken, chopped neatly into rows of timber waiting to be collected.

The door handle on the back of the van was slippery from the wet mist, but after a few tugs it freed itself, exposing behind the doors, wide frightened eyes from within. I didn't feel any pity, sadness or guilt, as to what these wretched creatures were experiencing. Try as I might, I couldn't find any compassion, 'maybe I should,' I thought to myself. But, no it did not come, nothing, my feelings numb.

The four by fours came to stop, I was aware of frantic movements to the side of me as the men all eight of them changed into green and brown camouflage gear, hats, coats, trousers and black thick leather boots.

'Have you let them go yet?' Bob called across the wooded clearing, his voice penetrating the cold damp air.

'No not yet,' I half whisper back to Bob, afraid to startle the creature within the van, 'they are waiting for their food and water first before their release.

'I must give them some strength before they go,' I think to myself, not daring to put too much emotion into my words afraid that the creatures within would pick up on a slither of weakness. I pulled the large box out from the behind the four by four vehicles and it slid over towards me with ease. I remove the packets and tore them open, pushing one of the contents through the bars sectioned off at the back. I had to take my hand away quickly for fear of being grabbed or bitten. I emptied water into the metal bowls, and listened to the noise as the food was torn apart.

I stepped back outside and looked around, the mist was clearing, weak sunrays tried to penetrate the mist but not quite managing it. I watched as steam rose up from the logs. I walked over and sat on the edge of one, green moss and fungi spouting from around the fallen trunk of a once grand tree. The wetness from the trunk unable to penetrate my green and brown jacket, waterproof hunting jacket, a hot cup of coffee was thrust into my hand, 'thanks,' I said, to Jim, whose smile seemed never to falter, and if anything looked like it had been surgical stitched onto his face.

'Good day for it,' Jim said, taking a bite out of a cheese roll, 'we should have quite a sport today, just the right conditions,' he said, as he looked around at the others, busying themselves with hot drinks.

'Yes a good day,' I replied, trying to muster as much enthusiasm as the others, but not quite managing it in my tone of voice. A cheese roll was handed to me, I could not make out by whom, the dark ski mask hiding most of their face. I shake my head 'no'; decline the food, the pit of my stomach too churned up to enjoy food.

Jim picking up on mood of apprehension and said, 'look I know it's your first time, but you will get use to it and maybe start to enjoy it, look over there, Bob loves it, lives for it in fact. Remember however you look at it or take the view of what is right or wrong, just remember it is tradition, part of our culture, it must live on.'

I nodded my head in agreement with him, and took a sip of the hot sweet liquid, 'I know you are right, but it just takes some getting used to.... the idea of all of this,' I said, my throat now burning from the boiling liquid, 'it's not something that I have grown up with. I mean not part of my childhood.'

Bob, leaned closer, his face set in a tight grimace, and said, 'we need to keep it going, can't lose it you know, all those demonstrations, about it not being right, we need to keep our ways alive,' he relaxed his face and smiled a very lop sided smile, and turned and walked back towards the others.

Jim beckoned for me to leave. I threw the remainder of the contents of my cup on the log, and stood up, and slowly walked over towards the driver's side of the dirty off white van. 'Ready,' he said, as he jumped up beside me, 'let's try and get through the rest of this godforsaken track,' he said, as I started up the engine. I turned the key and the engine purred into action, and slowly we inched our way further up the hill towards the thickest part of the woods, 'got to give them some chance,' he said, laughing, 'as it won't be much sport,' he snorted this time with a stifled laughter, unwound the window and spat.

I don't know why but I was being very careful with the cargo in the back, 'I didn't want to hurt them,' I thought to myself, but that was laughable with what was about to happen soon.

The wheels got stuck again, I revved and revved, mud and dirt splatter up over the back wheels, but no amount of throttle was going to shift it. 'Shit,' I said, as I desperately pushed my foot harder to the floor.

'It's not going anywhere at the moment,' Jim said, as he looked over his shoulder out of the window, 'we shall just have to let them go here, and come back with some wood to move it later.'

'We ...can't,' but my words had gone on deaf ears, Jim had already got out of the passenger door, and was moving at speed to the back.

Jim pulled on the handle and the van door opened, 'what a sorry lot we have in here,' he said peering in the van, 'no good to man or beast, this bloody lot. Must be coming to the last of the stock, need to search for more soon, have a look on that web site when I get back see if we can raise some more, what's it called again?' Jim asked more to himself than to me.

'You can't let them go here,' I protest, maybe a little too hard with a hint of desperation in my voice, because Jim threw a look towards my way a look that could render someone rigid to the spot in fear. I try again, a little harder this time, 'there isn't much shelter for them to hide.'

'No time to waste,' Jim said ignoring me, reaching to the shelf above the side door, and taking out his rifle, 'those protesters will be here soon. God knows how they have been finding our hunts. Don't want them filming us again, only 'chase the buggers' the law says now, but what's the fun in that I ask you? Always hunted with a rifle always, chased them, always hunted, been in my family for years, and those wimps, those protesters aren't going to change our ways.'

I looked at the younger one of the bunch, cowering at the back eyes wide open with freight, 'oh good got ourselves a pregnant one in the back. I do love a pregnant one, great prize,' Jim said, spitting on the floor once again. 'Right you take this lot,' he said, handing me a pile of red coats, 'take charge of them,' I placed the coats on the floor, careful not to get mud on them, they had been cleaned and stitched from the last hunt.

'Right you lot go on , get the hell out of here,' Jim said brandishing his rifle towards the back of the cage. I unlocked the cage and stood back, 'right you know the tradition, put those red coats on, and stand over there.' I watched as the creatures put the red coats on. 'Right now run you fuckers, run, you know the score,' Jim shouted.

I watched with a mixture of emotion as the group of five, four men and one woman put their red coats on. They stood rooted to the spot for a few minutes, with a crack of the whip; they were soon running towards the woods.

'Right,' Jim said, 'we give them the usual time, and then we hunt them. We need to get some more stock, that web site, yes, I remember, history part one, Dulvaston Fox Hunt; we need to purchase the prize the hunt master himself. They use to hunt, now they have become the hunted and the foxes, well the foxes are safe, the deer they are safe too.'

Dear Shelagh, Snow Storm on the M1

I rang my son Alex up the other evening, 'I am going past your place, is it ok to call in and see you both?' I asked Alex over the phone, 'I haven't seen you since the wedding in Cyprus. I held my breath, not sure what the response would be aware that Ellen ruled the house and what Ellen says, goes. 'Yes that would be great, call in and stay overnight,' Alex replied. 'Ok,' I said, 'I will arrive at five in the afternoon, then I won't outstay my welcome,' I stifled a nervous laugh, 'it would be good to see you both.' I added the both bit with my teeth gritted, and my face set in a grimace, because I hated that overbearing wife of his. 'I shall set off early on Monday, and make my way up to Grimsby so only one night, but it would be lovely to see you both, it has been a while now.'

I was off to my parents for Christmas the first time in five years, 'a nice change,' I thought to myself. The journey up country was a long and difficult route, and normally I drove up the A46 across country, avoiding as much as I could of the motorways. To visit my son, I would have to change my route and travel up through all motorways, adding another thirty miles to my journey, and possibly another hour. But, it was worth it to see him.

Sunday the twentieth was only a couple of days off, so I rang again to check that all was ok, and that I could still visit my son, and his answer was 'yes do come and stay.'

I took my car to the garage on the Thursday seventeenth of December, to have the cam belt fitted, and the wheel baring changed. Then I would be sure that my five year old Mazda would be up for the long journey. On route to the garage, I pulled into the petrol station, and filled the car, this would save me time, as soon as my car had been fixed, I would be all ready for the journey. I would only need to collect the car, load it up and then I would be off lunch time Sunday the twentieth December.

It was early afternoon on Thursday when I had the phone call from the garage, 'sorry but we have found a problem with your car, and we are waiting for the part to be delivered. It won't be ready now until Monday,' the mechanic said over the phone. I sucked in my breath and thought hard, 'I have to leave Sunday,' I replied, feeling worried, anxious even. I could not let Alex down. 'No problem,' the cheery voice over the end of the phone said, 'we have a car we can lend you.'

I was collected in the car by the mechanic that was to be my loan car over Christmas, a little white Peugeot, P registered, and the heater was stuck on hot, and there was no music system or radio. I liked to have radio four on whilst driving, it takes my mind off the miles and miles of tarmac that I need to travel on in order to get to my destination, it just makes driving that little bit more relaxing. 'Still it's a car that goes,' I thought as I sat next to the mechanic as we drove back to the garage so I could drop him off.

I filled the little white Peugeot with fuel and took it back home, then loaded it ready for my journey the next day. I would set off at twelve o'clock in time for about five. I sat down in front of the television and watched the news, 'extreme bad weather is set to cover the Midlands and the northern part of Britain Sunday evening,' the weatherman said, as I watched the bright blue colours dotted over the map of Britain, then little snow shower markers came up, they too were dotted over the map, this did not look good, finally in large red letters underneath the map, 'Weather Warning, do not travel unless absolutely necessary.'

'This is necessary travel,' I said to myself, 'well at least, I will miss the weather front,' I said out loud to the weather man, who had now disappeared behind more maps, 'I am going Sunday afternoon, not in the evening.'

On Saturday afternoon, I thought it a good idea to go and buy some chocolate and water just in case I got stuck in the storm. I sat behind the wheel of the little Peugeot and started it up. Nothing happened; the engine would not turn over. I tried for five to ten minutes desperate to get that little old car started but nothing happened. I rang the garage but no reply, and then I remembered being told that they were shut early on Saturday morning, ready for their Christmas dinner later that evening. The garage was closed, I was stuck.

I sat at my kitchen table and thought hard, what could I do? I had two cars full of fuel one on a ramp in a locked garage, and the other outside my front door, that was refusing to start up. I walked across to the hall window and looked out, there tucked up on the side of the grass verge was my old white Peugeot, R registered, my old car. It was still taxed and MOT until February, but not insured. It had not been moved for months, I had left it, neglected it in fact, thinking that I could no longer use such an old car for long journeys, which was why I bought the Mazda. I picked up the keys to my old car. I sat inside, and then placed the key in the engine and turned, nothing happened. This was not surprising since I had not been near the car for months. I tried a second time; it fired up, the engine turned over.

I ran inside the house, picked up my phone and dialled my insurance company. Ten minutes later I was insured and one hundred and sixty pounds lighter in my bank. I drove the car to the garage and filled up with diesel. I then drove back home, unloaded the little white Peugeot with all my Christmas parcels and boxes, into my old Peugeot, it was now ready, I was ready to go, three cars full of fuel and only one working.

Sunday the twentieth came, I took the dogs for a long walk, had some lunch, and checked my car once more, and then at twelve o'clock I was ready to leave. The sun was bright as I left my little village behind. I switched on the radio, channel four kicked into life; I was ready to drive the miles and miles of black tarmac towards Ilkeston to visit my son.

I was making good time, the sky was clear, the weak December sun shone through the window of my car. I had cleared Bristol and was near my usual turn off junction nine

Tewkesbury, the A46 which I would normal take if going straight to my parents, but instead of turning off I drove past and further up on the M5, towards the M42 turn off. I was listening to a good play on the radio, and before long I saw the sign for M1, relief swept over me, this had been a good run, and I was only about half an hour from my destination, Alex's home.

My attention now turned to the Christmas gift bag on the front seat next to me. 'I hope they like their Christmas presents,' I thought, as I looked over and caught a glance of the neatly wrapped packages inside the gift bag. I had taken a lot of time pondering over what to buy my son and his wife. This would be the first Christmas present to my son. The last time I had bought him a present was when he was three years old, I had not seen him again until recently.

I had splashed out on more than I could afford, but it was worth it, my son was worth it, the large bottle of good quality French brandy was wrapped in red and silver Christmas paper, and next to it was a large box of Thornton's chocolates for his wife, a small bottle of red wine, and bubble bath were my other gifts, 'I hope they like them,' my thoughts were suddenly interrupted with a loud shrill from my mobile phone sitting next to me on the front seat.

I leaned over and switched it to hands free speaker. 'Hello,' I called out towards the phone. 'Its Alex here,' came a voice on the other end, 'we have snow here,' he continued, 'it's snowing.'

I looked out of the window clear skies in front of me, and I was twenty miles away. 'It's not snowing here,' I laughed, 'bright blue clear skies here, I am only twenty miles from you Alex, won't be long now, just coming along the A42 quite near the M1.' There was silence on the phone, 'hello, are you there?' I called out.

Alex's voice came over the loud speaker, 'well it's snowing hard here covering the ground,' he said sounding faint now. 'Look Alex, I can't hear you properly, how about I come off at the next service station and I ring you back?' I waited for a few seconds, and then he replied, 'ok.'

I drove on looking for the next turn off, the sky was clear of clouds, not a single snow cloud in sight, 'this is strange,' I thought to myself, 'I can't see any signs of snow.' The blue service sign came into view, 'nine miles to the next service station.' I looked down at the clock on the dash board of the car, 'three thirty,' the sun was quickly setting behind me, I could see its tips of orange glow in the rear view mirror, the blue sky quickly turning to a display of reds, orange and small puffs of white clouds, that gave out a pink glow.

I indicated, to turn off for the service station, this was the last one before the M1. Alex only lived a few miles from the M1 in-between Nottingham and Derby, my journey was nearly over. I parked the car, and picked up the phone and dialled Alex's number. 'Hi,' he said, 'it's still snowing here,' came the reply. 'Well its clear here Alex,' I said, silence, not sure what else to say, then I added, 'I am not far from you now, could do with a nice cup of tea when I arrive there,' I reply laughing. 'You won't make it here,' he said again, his voice now had the tone of someone who was acutely embarrassed. I pushed him further, 'what do you mean I won't make it there?' I asked now sounding confused, 'I am only five miles away.' A long silence followed, I heard him take in a huge breath, 'I mean it is a few inches deep,' he replied.

I looked around me; the sky was clear even though at ten past four dusk was setting in quickly, this being one day off from the shortest day of the year. 'You won't get here,' he said, once more, this time with a strong sense of urgency to his voice. 'Oh shit,' I said sounding hugely disappointed, and totally confused, 'what the hell should I do?' not able to disguise the tiredness getting into the tone of my voice. The silence on the other end of the phone was embarrassingly long; it was too long for comfort, until I was given no choice but to reply to it. 'I suppose I had better press on then,' I say, not sure what else to say. I could hear the sigh of relief from the voice at the other end of the phone. 'Ok that would be a good idea. Bye,' Alex said.

I flipped the phone onto the passenger's seat, stared hard and long out of the window, confusion raked my brain, then lightness filtered through like a sieve. 'I get it,' I said out aloud to my doggy companions on the back seat, 'I fucking get it, he doesn't want me there, she doesn't want me there, I am not wanted,' my own son does not want me.

My head slowly turns to the Christmas gift set, all neatly wrapped up with a loving gift tag attached to the red and silver gift bag. I look at the gift bag, but I can't see it, it is blurred, out of focus, that is until I rub my eyes with my sleeve, then it comes back into focus but only briefly, then it disappears again. The tears are salty as they slip between my lips into my mouth.

I start the engine and drive slowly out of the service station and back onto the A42, and for the next ten minutes the car is on auto pilot as I replay the conversation over and over again in my head. I indicate and swing out left and into the lane for the M1. Five miles onto the busy motorway, I see it; I see the huge black cloud that dominates the skyline in front of me. I have now swung a left and was heading north, and there in front of me was a frighteningly roll of dark clouds moving straight into my path, or was I moving towards them? It was nasty. This was the weatherman's warning, and I had no choice but to drive towards it. I had come too far to turn back.

It came in quick both at the same time, the darkness and the snow, it fell together, no day light and no vision as the thick white snowflakes covered my front window. I was nearly driving blind. I slowed down to twenty miles an hour, the road was busy, and on all side of me was traffic each one of us crawling along in a blizzard. 'This is bloody scary,' I call out to the dogs.

I had fifteen minutes of difficult driving when I saw the sign, that large blue motorway sign and in big bold letters the word Ilkeston was written. This should have been my turn off. I blinked back the tears, as I tried to concentrate on the road ahead, which was now only visible at a few yards, my only guidance was the other traffic ahead of me their dazzling red and orange lights from the vehicles, their braking lights, hazard warning lights.

The snow was piling up fast on the road, which turned to slush and ice; the quick movement of the wipers were no match for the thick fast snowflakes driven in with the howling wind. 'This is dangerous,' I thought to myself, as I braked hard and brought my speed down to ten miles an hour, a lorry was inches in front of me to my left, I was now somehow stuck in the outside lane, I wanted to move back, get into the far side lane, get out of this heavy traffic with visibility down to an extremely low level this was a driver's worse nightmare.

I glanced in my rear view mirror, I could only see glows of lights, nothing tangible, nothing solid, just a haze of lights, 'Christ,' I said aloud, 'I need to move over.' I indicated and held my breath I edge my way out to the middle lane, then again to the inside lane, hoping and praying that the vehicle behind would notice my intentions and slow down and give me space.

I slid into the inside lane, near the hard shoulder, and followed the haze of lights through wipers that were working incredible hard, desperately trying to brush aside the fast flowing snowflakes. 'Shit, shit,' I cried out aloud, the tears welled up once more, my cheeks stung with the salty tears, the blurry lights of the vehicles in front increased with blurriness as my eyes welled up with tears spilling with ease down my face. 'What sort of son sends his own mother out in this weather?' I shout out aloud, as I slam on my brakes as the vehicle in front slammed theirs on. 'What have I done so wrong?' I whisper to myself, as the snow gathers with pace on the overworked wipers. 'Bloody families' I cry.

My sleeve wipes away another salty tear, and I glance back across at my gift bag, the tag swinging back and forwards with the movements of the car. 'Not wanted should now be written on the tag, these gifts were not wanted, I wasn't wanted.' I brake suddenly as I stop only inches away from the white van in front of me. My blurred vision combined with my overworked wipers, was creating a dangerous situation on the roads. 'I will be lucky if I get out of here alive,' I think, 'then maybe that might just be the answer to my hurt. No more pain, nothing, all this will be gone.'

I ease back on the accelerator, instead just lightly touching it with my foot. 'This is madness,' I think, 'just pure madness. The snow had worsen, visibility had turned more to luck than judgement, 'wouldn't put a cat out in this,' I say to myself, 'but you can put your own mother out.' Self pity swamps me; I wallow in self pity, hurt, and anger, and think to the moment my son is told his mother has died. 'Road accident,' the police officer would say. 'That will teach him,' I think in my own messed up mind.

I look up, the M18 has come into view, I indicate and turn off, five miles up the motorway the snow has eased off, the traffic has eased, conditions return to near normal. I look back at the gift bag the tag with 'Happy Christmas lots of love mum' written on. The first Christmas since he was three, 'not wanted,' I think, and drive on.

White Snake

It was a beautiful morning. It was six thirty and late September the colours on the trees had not yet changed, autumn was late arriving, it was an Indian summer. The walk takes me up across a ploughed field, and then up to a small cider apple orchard a young one, then to the top ridge, where I can take a left to keep on the public footpath, or right that takes me along the ridge and passes three large fields. A row of trees and bushes are on the left, the trees are bent at an angle from the fierce winter winds.

This morning I took a right turning, and walked along the hard ground, rain had not come for over a month, and the earth was solid, cracked, and hard walking. The dogs ran beside me, stopping and sniffing the air, then walking and running on ahead. I stopped and looked behind me, the sun was trying to rise but slowly now that winter was creeping in, and a thin layer of mist lay over the distant lands, the fields, the trees, and out towards the sea.

I turned around and carried on walking; I had to watch my feet, as the ground was uneven, rocky and rubble thrown over from the heavy plough that had recently gone over the soil. I took a minute to look up and just ahead a glittering object, shimmering a few feet away. I walked closer, not able to quite make out what it might be, the object came into view, and I stood rooted to the spot.

A silver snake lay curled up on the ground, its scales the colour of pearls, glisten in the light, as the weak sun's rays caught it. I moved slowly closer, only my natural instinct is to freeze, I have a fear of snakes, or anything that slithers and slides, and usually my feet tingle, my hands grow clammy. But, not this time, this beautiful creature, lay basking in the tepid warm sun, not much warmth so early in the morning, but just enough.

I was now only a few feet away, and could see clearly this beautiful graceful creature, no bigger than a few feet long, with a slender sleek body, that lay half coiled up. The snake raised its head, and looked at me, its hypnotic eyes, that looked deep into the soul, its eyes burning into my eyes.

I looked back, not afraid, my hands not tingling, and not wanting to run. I moved slowly around the creature, so as not to startle it. It moved its head and followed my direction. I was now on the other side of the snake and ready to walk along the ridge; my two dogs had crossed over the field and were waiting by the gate. I was surprised that they hadn't noticed the snake. 'Had they seen it?' I thought to myself, 'with its colour, it couldn't have been missed.' But, no my two dogs were waiting by the gate on the other side of the snake.

I walked on a few feet passed it, I stopped and turned around. I blinked as the sun now dazzled my vision, and peered hard at the ground, but it was gone. There wasn't a snake there anymore. I walked back, the grass were it had laid, was clearly not disturbed, instead, it was as though there had been nothing lying in the spot. I placed my hand down on the grass, it was cold, but then a shiny object caught my eye, it was a glistening scale like a mother of pearl, lying in the grass. I bent down and picked it up, it slipped between my fingers and search as I tried, I couldn't find it again.

That was this morning, had it all been a dream? I had been suffering from my depression, my hurt and my anxiety, so was it my mind playing tricks on me? I had been thinking about the snake all day, all the way back from my walk, wondering where it had come from. Was it an escaped exotic creature from the big house down the lane? Was it a rare creature that I had seen, now gone back into hiding? The big question though, was I going mad?

Later in the afternoon, I went out again with the dogs, this time it is a short walk, not far just down to the bridge. It was warm, unusually warm for the time of year. Instead of a heavy jumper to keep out the autumn chill, I wore a light tee-shirt over my thin blue trousers. I placed my sunglasses over my eyes to shield them from the harsh glare of the midday sun.

I had only got as far as the bottom of the road when the sun burned down on me, my skin hot, wet from the perspiration. I crossed over the road and walked the few hundred yards to the bridge, the dogs were still tired from their morning walk. The leads were slack in my hand. I stood on the edge of the bridge and looked down into the shallow water, normally it is a swirling torrent from the swollen rivers on the moors, but today there was barely a trickle of water.

For some reason, unknown to me, I walked down the footpath next to the bridge, and through a gap in the hedge. The water in the river was clear, sparkling, unlike the muddy mass of dirt and filth dragged along the hedge banks where litter has been discarded. I was about to turn around when something out of the corner of my eye caught my attention. The dogs were busy paddling around in the water, drinking and sniffing the edges, so with my hands now free I scrambled over some rocks exposed from the river bank.

My foot slipped, and for a split second I lost my balance, but with my hands waving madly around in the air I managed to steady myself. I grabbed an overhanging branch and pulled myself up and over the rocks; I was now some way down the river bank, which is normally under water.

I noticed it again, it was shiny. A spider's web so beautifully woven, that at first it did not appear to be a spider's web at all, but a delicate lace cloth, this is not what caught my eye, but what was inside the spider's web, a shiny, black stone, the size of a walnut. The stone was so deep, and dark, that at first it appeared to be a jewel of some kind. I stood in awe of this object, never had I seen such a thing in a spider's web.

I turned and stepped back my foot slipped and I landed in the icy cold water. I called the dogs and walked away. I was puzzled what was that shiny stone doing in a spider's web? How had it got there? Who put it there? It definitely wasn't a fly; it was a stone, a rock, or even metal. I had not touched it for fear of it breaking the delicate web, and all I had to go on was the look, it definitely looked like a precious jewel.

I had a relaxing afternoon, I spent the time, reading and sipping hot milky coffee, in the garden, in the shade. I looked down at the bottom of the garden, my chickens were enjoying the sun, they were sunning themselves. The dogs were sprawled out on the grass asleep.

I must have dozed off for a while, when I opened my eyes the sun had started to slip behind the clouds, daylight shorter now, the chill in the air made me shiver. I slowly stood up and stretched then gathered my cup and walked into the house.

As twilight slowly ebbed its way into the skies, I took my coat off the hook and took the dogs out for their last walk. This is a very short walk, just around the few houses where I live. There is no street light, and without a torch with me, I had to walk quickly before darkness set in.

At first I thought they were birds flying around, looking for a branch to settle down on for the night, but they were too quick for birds, as they darted in and out of the trees, swooping low. 'These are bats,' I thought to myself. I don't mind bats; in fact I quite like them, an air of mystic as they dart around in the dark.

I was on my home when something brushed my hair, it was quite dark now, very little natural daylight left, in fact I had left it later than usual to walk the dogs, I had dozed longer than I had intended. I felt it again, but could see little, my hair moved; it flew out from my face. It was though an invisible hand swept passed me, brushed me with finger tips, gentle, not rough. 'Was it the wind?' I thought to myself, but the night was airless, not even a light breeze. 'Was it a branch?' I said aloud hurrying my feet along, which felt like blocks of lead.

The night was pitch black, the clouds had covered the moon, and then again my hair blew out, like an electric shock. The clouds parted, a spiral of moonlight shone down, my eyes growing accustomed to the light, I peered hard into the night. A whisper of hair flew away from my face, it hung outwards, strange and airy, then I caught the culprit, a bat. But, this was no ordinary bat, this was a white bat. A pure white bat, had caught my hair, it gently tugged at it, playing with it, catching it with its claws, as it swooped low. 'It is playing,' I say aloud into the darkness. I am not afraid.

Three strange events took place today, not everyday occurrences, but strange things, strange sights. 'Was it madness?' I ask myself, 'did it happen?' 'What is real and what is not?' I asked myself, as I look out into the darkness from the safety of my bedroom. The moon has gone now, the thick clouds covering the ray of light. I yawn, I am tired, I stretch my arms, my bed looks welcoming, sleep, I must sleep. I take one last look from my bedroom window, a quarter of moon, lights up my garden step, I look down, I gasp I step back, I look down again, but it has gone, that figure in black, that face, that white face staring back at me. A face, so white, but the eyes so dark, as though no eyes at all.

Chapter two

I took the same route that I had taken yesterday, only today, the mist was hanging low, so low in fact that my coat was wet with the heavy dew. I walked up panting past the orchard, the apples hanging heavy and low on the laden branches. My breathing was always difficult when climbing up steep slopes but especially so with a heavy mist, their air damp and moist.

Finally as I stood at the green sign post pointing left to the public footpath, only I took the right instead and walked towards where I had seen the white snake yesterday. My footsteps were quicker than normal, and so was my breathing, my heart was also banging against my chest. I looked down at the place where I had seen the snake.

There was no snake, not even a sign of one, but just to the left tucked away under a bramble, a large overhanging blackberry bush, lying on the ground on its side was a rabbit, it was a young rabbit, its eyes wide open, dried blood trickling from the shot wound on the side of its head. It saddens me to see an animal killed for the sake of killing, for sport, not for food, just for fun. I walked on, my heart sunk by the unnecessary killing of a young defenceless animal.

I reached the gate, my two dogs stood wagging their tails their tongues hanging out, and we walked on. Behind the gate lay another rabbit, it too had been shot, left by the side of the high Devon bank running along the edge of the field. Further on just past the small crop of trees, three more rabbits lay dead, they had been killed, shot, thrown down by their burrow.

Unable to continue my walk I turned around and walked past the dead rabbits, their lifeless bodies lying rotting in the sun that was now rising, no more would they see the sun, no more would they feed on the corn, they were gone.

I walked home; anger hit me, anger at how killing could be fun. I tried to push my anger to the back of my mind, and fed my dogs. I too then went inside the house, cooked my porridge and tried to function on my daily activities, ones that we need to do, cook for ourselves, clean, and wash, it is the same wherever, we are, we can't function without so many daily chores, it is a necessity of life. We are bound by routine each and every one of us, no matter how hard we try to escape it, because daily routine comes in the way of sleeping, waking, and feeding ourselves. We are each and every one of us creatures of habit.

Routine for me was to walk again down to the bridge, this is the short walk. The river was barely a foot deep in some parts; the rains hadn't fallen for months. I was drawn down to the same spot that I had gone to yesterday. I stood on the rock and with my hands waving around balanced myself in a position to look across at the spider's web, but it too had gone. I jumped down off the rock, fell and landed my hand touching something soft under the grassy bank.

I parted the branches and there lying underneath, its body still warm was a deer, a young deer, it too had been shot, thrown over the bridge. I sat with the deer stroking its warm body, why it was still warm I have no idea, because it had obviously lain dead for some time. I stood up and wiped my face, my dogs were in the water, 'strange' I thought, 'why hadn't they picked up its smell?'

I walked back home, the sun beating hard down on my face, sweat dripping from my body, it was unbelievably warm on this late autumn day. The sadness that filled my heart with the deaths of those animals stayed with me.

I went outside and sat under the tree, a glass of cold freshly squeezed lemon juice in my hand. I took a sip, and placed the glass on the green plastic table, and sat back in the hard metal green chair, and shut my eyes.

It was cool when I woke up, my eyes were sore from the redness of crying earlier, my back ached from the angle of sitting in the chair with my head resting on the table. How long I had been there I was not sure, but it must have been a good few hours because I was stiff.

The evening light was fading. I walked into the house, picked up the dogs leads and hooked them up. There wasn't much time before the night set into darkness, 'the cloudless night might give some moonlight,' I thought, as I set off down the road for our last walk before bed.

I felt something against my foot, I stopped and bent down and touched the object, the ray of light shone down and I was able to see the dead badger lying by the side of the road. I moved it slowly to the side.

There were no bats tonight, the air was still, just enough light to light my way through the back road. There was enough light to make out a shape on the side of the road, it was the size of a dog, perhaps it was a dog, I thought to myself, as I came nearer to it, but the long bushy tail, was not that of a dog, it was a young fox, much the same age as the badger.

These deaths, I thought to myself, 'why?' but there was no answer, I couldn't understand. There was no white bat, in fact any bats tonight.

The sadness of the deaths hit me as I walked up the stairs to my bed, 'was I going mad?' I thought to myself, 'perhaps I didn't see the animals, maybe it is my mind playing tricks. It's not real, none of it is real.' The moon shone down on the garden, I could see the entire garden tonight, and it was a full moon, big and bright. I stood for quite some time at the window of my bedroom, reluctant to sleep, my nightmares had increased recently, so sleep was not welcoming, only a necessity to keep me from tiredness.

I turned around and walked to my bed, no figure tonight, so maybe it was my mind playing tricks on me. I had to walk back to the window just one more time, just to be sure. I stood and looked out, there was no figure tonight, 'a relief,' I said to myself, 'thank goodness.' I was just about to turn away when my eyes caught sight of something in the garden, it took some time for them to focus, but when at last they did, I gasp out loud, the figure was slowly walking up the garden. It had a long black coat, it hung loosely around its tall thin frame, unable to tell whether it were male or female because of the hood pulled up. The face looked up at the window, the black eyes met mine, they were not hard to miss in the white face.

I should have been afraid. I should have run, but then my feet wouldn't move, I was rooted to the spot. The figure lifted off the ground, it floated closer to the window, I leaned nearer. I needed to see the face. I must see the face. But, the cloud covered the moon, it was a black cloud, and the moon was once again hidden, sending the garden into blackness, deep blackness, and thick like velvet.

I was too unhappy to be afraid. The deaths of the animals hurt me more than my children; my children hurt me, but not as much as those deaths of the animals, pointless deaths.

That figure, it could not hurt me, nothing more could hurt me when I was already hurting so much inside? I turned over in bed and close my eyes waiting for the nightmares to start up, because they would soon, they always did. 'None of it made sense,' I thought to myself, as I lay in bed waiting for sleep to take over me. My life was so full of hurt, deep rooted pain within me never leaving always with me, walking beside me hand in hand in life, and when at times the pain eases just a little, not much, then just as it goes, the pain that is, then something nasty rears its ugly head, hits me in the guts, like looking at 'road kill' on a routine walk. I never did get over my journey north for Christmas.

Why can't others share this planet? Why do we take it upon ourselves to destroy what is around us? Life and Death so much, hand in hand, narrow road, famers taking aim, guns fired, death and destruction amidst a planet full of beauty.

I take my step ladder and climb up onto the roof, and write in bold lettering in thick white paint, 'beam me up Scotty', this place is shit.

You shop we drop

The early morning mist shrouded the lush green valley below, nestled between the tree lined hills. The watery orange glow peeped through the patches of mist as the sun's rays worked their way through the tree's branches, not long and the whole valley would be bathed in sunlight. Now, in the early hours of the morning, two chestnut-coloured deer stood majestically; surrounded by red Poppies. The red Poppy flowers moved as though dancing to the tune of the breeze, and yellow ripening corn, bowed and swayed, touched gently by the passing air on the valley floor.

In the distance small brown dots sat perfectly still, nibbling on dew tipped grasses, white dots bobbed away towards shrubs at the end of the field, the whites of their tails a contrast against the backdrop of the brown field, recently ploughed, on the far side of the river.

The tips of the dark green trees, pushed through the mist bathed in the early morning sun, like a submarine beginning to rise through the grey ocean waters. Buzzards circle high above the tips of the trees, catching the thermals, their wings stretched out, they rise and fall like a kite with an invisible string. It's the peace that catches you, nature in tune with nature, no sign of bumbling mankind, he's not arrived, the valley a safe haven.

The peace is shattered: a rumbling sound is heard, the rabbits take cover, the deer run, and the birds take flight. A yellow machine makes its way across the valley, white vans arrive, and men in fluorescent jackets, armed with clipboards, march across the fields. A line is drawn up the yellow machine comes forward with its mechanical jaws wide open, then with one fell swoop it's gone: the field has been transformed into black tarmac, white lines neatly drawn, a shining black car park lies in its place.

The shrubs are ripped out, bird's homes destroyed, rabbits with nowhere to go but under the wheels, their small bodies crushed into the roads. A fine building made of steel and glass proudly stands in the corner of the valley, it glitters and shines under the midday sun, the tall white pole stands proudly at the edge of the road, a blue and white Tesco flag flutters gently in the breeze.

A small brown deer rigid with fear stands in the middle of the road, not sure where to go, the large thundering articulated lorry catches the deer as if it were a paper bag, and tosses it to the side... You Shop We Drop the logo on the lorry reads, as it sweeps past the deer's small frail body; a crushed, lifeless, un-mourned heap by the side of the road.

Dear Shelagh, An Important Lunch

It was one of those days when things were suppose to go right, and if they did not I would be in trouble. It was Sunday and I was meeting my daughter for lunch. This is an important meal because we had not spoken to each other for months, we had a fallen out over her wedding. But, at last, I had managed to get us both together to talk.

Now Sundays are usually John days. The day when he comes over and we go to the little cafe in Branford Speke, run by Sue, who only does it as a hobby. The food is locally sourced and freshly cooked, not a lot of choice in fact only two choices, roast beef and vegetables, or the vegetarian lunch, with a choice of sweets, usually plum crumble, trifle, or treacle tart, not much choice but all freshly cooked.

I shall be taking my daughter to Sue's for lunch today, and I phone up and book a table, 'a table for two at twelve outside please,' I said to Sue. I was anxious that my daughter might not like my choice of venue for our meeting, but it was in the country, peaceful and good food.

Sunday arrived and I leave my house at eleven thirty which allows plenty of time to arrive at the café only five miles away, but five miles down the little country lanes around Devon. I park my car some way up the hill near my daughter's flat, there is no parking outside, and I walk up the path to the old Victorian house and ring the bell.

Heather smiles as she opens the door, her long blond hair freshly washed hangs around her shoulders, her slender wrists wear beads, pretty coloured bracelets, delicate gold bangles dangle from her right wrist, and rings, lots of pretty stoned, coloured rings. She's wearing a long flowing skirt, a white lace blouse, low flat green shoes, and a scarf; a soft silk green and red scarf loosely tied around her neck. 'Give me a minute,' she says, 'can you come in please and wait.' I follow her down the long corridor and into the brightly decorated living room.

I sit down on the red sofa bed, and look around the room: the Buddhist statues decorate the fireplace, incense sticks, recently burnt, dangle out of candle holders, Asian carpets hang on the wall, the windows have white fluffy fairy lights hanging down, the room is a mixture of modern and bohemian style.

'Thanks for the eggs,' my daughter said, as she takes the carton of eggs, laid by my chickens. She carries them into the kitchen and then hands me a bag, full of empty egg boxes, 'these are for you,' she says, 'I've been saving them up.' I thank my daughter for the egg boxes. I stand up and we walk back to the car. The time is now twelve o'clock, we are late.

'Nice car,' she says, as she gets into the blue Mazda. 'Oh this isn't mine, it is a friend's car I have borrowed,' I say to her, 'he has lent it to me.' Heather does not say anything, only looks: it is that look. We arrive at the café at ten past twelve, not too late. 'You're upstairs,' Sue says. Heather looks my way, 'oh I would much prefer to eat outside,' my daughter said, 'it's such a nice warm day. ' 'No problem,' Sue says, 'I forgot you were booked outside, please follow me.'

Heather stands looking around the tiny cobbled courtyard; a garage, at the end, has four tables inside, the garage door is wide open. The patio area, tiny, has many potted plants against the walls. I step over the plants, and sit down at the table, but it rocks: it's uneven on the stones. I try to shift it around, but the table is a heavy iron one, difficult to move; it takes some pulling and shoving, until I moved it a couple of inches. I sit down, but now it is worse than ever.

I pull and push again, back to where it was. 'Have you quite finished?' Heather asks, raising her eyebrows at me. The sun is now in my eyes, I squint and can't see, so I stand up to move my chair over a bit, but I lose my balance on the cobbled stones, and fall onto the pot plant which crashes into the wall; dirt and soil scattered all over the place. I lean over and pick it up. I take a peep at my daughter's face, it is set in stone: but I can't help myself, and I laugh. Not a good move.

I steady the pot plant, and sit down facing my daughter. 'Well, have you quite finished now?' she asks in a tone that a mother might use to scold a child. 'Yes, thank you, I have quite finished now,' I reply, but I am smiling, aware that my smile may appear fixed and lopsided. I am nearly losing the plot, and slowly descending into hysterics. I scold myself, 'be serious now,' I think to myself.

We order our food, and then we sit and talk, every day conversation, about Heather's new job. But, then I notice her looking to her left at the wall, a small hole is near her ear, and inside the hole is a spider peeping out. Heather has a fear of spiders bordering on extreme phobia. The food arrives, but the hole is more interesting than the food.

She keeps staring at the hole, and nudges her chair away from it. 'About my wedding,' she says. My heart drops, 'oh no, not the wedding,' I think to myself, 'anything but the wedding.' 'I would like to know how much you can afford towards it?' she asked, glancing at the hole in the wall. 'I thought you could pay for the wedding dress, the flowers and make the cake,' she said, and then takes a mouthful of her vegetarian meal, and looks again at the hole.

'That should be ok,' I say. 'Good,' Heather said, 'thanks that will be helpful. I also thought that since my father and his wife are not coming to the wedding ceremony, perhaps you could come to that and then leave at six, so that my father can come to the evening reception.' I finish my food, and push my plate to the side.

I did not say anything, there was nothing I could say because, if I had done, the meal would be finished and a row started. Besides which, Heather's attention is now fully engrossed elsewhere: towards the spider's hole from which now protrude an ever increasing number of long black hairy legs, and then suddenly my daughter quickly jumps up nearly knocking her chair over, and heads quickly for the door. I pay for our meal and drive her home.

I have just written a letter to my daughter, explaining that I am not happy about the wedding arrangement, when my mobile phone rings. It is Heather; she wants to know how much I will be paying towards the wedding. 'I have written you a letter,' I reply over the phone, 'because we cannot talk.' 'What do you mean we cannot talk,' she said, 'of course we can talk over the phone.' I take a deep breath, a moment silence passes, and then I go for it, 'well, look, I am not happy about leaving at six o'clock, I do not think it is fair: I did not get to go to Alex's wedding reception and now I will not be allowed to come to yours.' The silence at the other end was long, so long I thought she had put the phone down on me, when she said slowly, 'well since you will not compromise' and then put the phone down on me, and all that was left in my ear was a buzzing of an unused phone line.

That was four months ago, I have had no contact with my daughter since, she does not want to know to me. She has ignored my text messages pleading with her to talk. So the moral of the story, do not believe anyone who says they can talk, when clearly they cannot, especially when they pretend to be a non materialistic Buddhist, bloody families.

Dear Shelagh About my Night in a Police Cell

I lay down on the thin blue mattress. There was nothing else to do but stare at the ceiling. I knew I was being watched, and even though my immediate reaction was to scream and hammer at the locked door, I fought the impulse to do such a thing.

'No, don't draw attention to yourself. Just act normal,' I thought to myself, 'act normal, even though my reason for being here was anything but normal.'

I did let the tears slip down my face, that was a normal reaction, and I was unafraid to cry. I didn't just cry, after a few seconds of tears slipping down my cheeks, I let go and then whoosh a river burst its banks like most rivers on a thoroughly wet bank holiday afternoon. I sobbed uncontrollably, aware of my shoulders heaving up and down, my hands futilely wiping away wet patch after wet patch, and with no handkerchief, I had no choice but to use the thin white woolly blanket. I knew I was being watched on the overhead monitors, 'but let them watch,' I thought.

After what seemed like hours, I had no idea of the time, I pressed the speaker buzzer, next to the door, 'can I go to the ladies please?' I ask, very politely aware of my politeness, hoping this would go in my favour, 'and may I have the lights dimmed?'

A voice void of emotion returned with a short reply, 'I will get someone to take you to the toilets,' and then the lights went dim. I lay back and waited, and waited, my thoughts running all over the place like eggs running over a frying pan, with maybe a hint of a solid form resembling something like scramble eggs, coming together at the last second.

'Why was I here?' I kept asking myself over and over again, 'where did it all go wrong?' If I had a map of my past, my history, I would spread it out, and take a pin, and the pin would be placed hard down, so hard that it would go through the paper. The pin would never be removed again, and at that point, I thought to myself, listening to the heavy booted footsteps, dragging a protesting male voice to the cell opposite mine, 'sleep it off, you will be charged in the morning,' the police officer's gruff voice shouted above the slurred yelling din.

'That point,' I mulled over, my thoughts gathering pace once again, the scrambled mess assembling some sort of realisation, of where it all went so badly wrong. 'Ah yes that point that would be Hillsea Boarding School. The school that took away my childhood, robbed me of my life. That school were acts of abuse went on for years, hidden from view, under the radar so to speak, forgotten by the School Inspectors according to The Telegraph. That would be the point where the pin went sharply, firmly, even crossly into the map. Not angrily stabbed, besides what was the point of anger, or even bitterness? What was done was done. I was damaged, that was damaged beyond repair.'

I felt my eyes well up once again, a feeling of feeling sorry for myself engulfing me. I sniffed, rubbed my nose, and sat up. There were footsteps approaching my cell door.

'You wanted to go the toilet?' a young female police officer asked. I nodded and followed her the short distance, and was shown into a small cubicle, with no door. She stood by the cubical watching me squat and pee. No dignity here, I was beyond human.

Finished I was taken back to my cell, and the heavy door slammed behind me, stirring the occupant opposite, a drunken incomprehensible mutterings echoed around the prison cells.

I sat on my thin blue mattress, 'I am here because of pain,' I thought to myself as I lay down on the hard cold surface, 'the unfairness of it all, the unjustness, me a product of my childhood at the hands of adults in charge of me, 'childhood?' I questioned, maybe out loud this time, because my thoughts ran together once more, fast flowing spilling outwards, as I remembered my past, those days of sitting huddled outside my in-law's house in the early hours of the morning, rocking backwards and forwards my arms tight around me, stabbing, throbbing pain within, as my cries for my children, my two young babies went unheard, a thin mist of dawn cold vapour blew out from between my chattering teeth, another pin in the map of my past, and a point in my life where death was a welcoming presence.

It was in the early hours of the morning when the heavy door opened, and a small figure in a suit appeared beside two police officers. 'Miss Holmes?' the suit asked.

I nodded, my face redden with crying, and so too were my eyes, and as for my nose, well that was full of crying sniffles, blocked, and snuffled.

'Yes,' I snuffled.

'This way please,' said one of the police officers, again a voice void of emotion, where do they learn this emotionless voice. I followed the suit, bare foot, my shoes removed on entry to the police station. The two police officers close behind me, just in case I was to make a bolt for it, 'but would I?'

The room I was shown into was sparse, a small table, two white plastic chairs, and a sink. 'So what brought you here Miss Holmes?' The suit asked. The police officers looked on from just outside the door.

I looked at one, who was looking at me, and I answered the suit's question. 'If you have a daughter, who is getting married, then may I suggest you book yourself a room in here, a cell like mine,' I said.

I felt this was not quite the response the suit thought he would get, but he got it, because that was the bizarre truth of this whole sorry incident.

'It's like this,' I said, not crying anymore, but trying to get a grip on this ridiculous situation, 'my daughter is getting married on the first of May, and I asked who was going to be best man, thinking she would have my father, her grandfather or even her brother, so I was taken aback when she said, it was going to be Sam's father, her soon to be father in-law. I suppose I got quite upset about the whole marriage thing. Relations between my daughter and me are strained at the best of times, in fact I liken my daughter to someone who is surrounded by eggshells, and woe betide anyone who treads on one. I suppose I just felt that I had not been good enough for her. You know the sort a single mother, living in a council house, five times married, with her half brothers that have only recently come into our lives,' I said breathless, spilling a part of my sorry life out to a stranger in a suite in the middle of the night in a police cell.

'Go on,' said the suit, wondering how this would bring me into a police cell in the middle of the night.

'Well I have been under a lot of pressure just recently, my nerves have been frayed, fraught even, and my stress levels shot through the roof, and all to do with my lost boys. My two young sons who were taken away from me when babies,' I said, choosing to miss out the kidnapping bit, in case this went against me, 'and only recently came back into my life, but then finding my son's like strangers.

'Your daughter rang the police telling them that you suffer from borderline personality disorder, and that you were going to kill yourself, and when they could not get you on the phone they feared the worse,' the suit said. 'I am sorry you had to come into the police station and into a police cell, but there was no room at the mental health hospital, they were full.'

'I am fine now,' I lied, taking a deep breath and wiping away my tears. 'Are you?' the suit asked.

'Yes, I am perfectly ok, and so sorry to have caused yourself and the police any unnecessary worry about my mental health state. I should not have got upset over the wedding arrangement, but my daughter wants the perfect day, and if I just show any sign of disagreement with her arrangements then she flares up, but unfortunately my reaction to her reaction is to either shout or threaten to kill myself, but this time I did not scream at her instead threatened to kill myself, but I am fine now.'

The suit made notes, the police officers shifted their feet, and the airy silence of the police station was quietness closing in. My freedom was now on the line, my only hope was had I done enough to convince those who needed convincing that I was telling the truth when in fact I was lying, and I still felt like ending it all. I did not want to be locked up again, not in the mental health hospital where criminals have better treatment then the mentally ill. Stripped, searched and drug tested, thrown into a stinking, filthy, room with lights switched on every hour, every bit of your last piece of dignity as a living human being shredded. You are nothing, no one with any rights. Even a criminal has more rights than someone sectioned. I know I have seen it happen when it was me the professional on the other side, as a mental health social worker.

'Well ok,' the suit said, then a very long pause, too long. Papers are shuffled around, more ink scribbling, more notes, and then finally, 'well you can go now.' 'Thank you,' I said.

It was seven o'clock when I was dropped off at home by the police, my dogs were howling, my cats were hungry, and my chickens were protesting at being shut up in their coup.

I made a cup of tea, had a bite to eat, hooked up the two dogs on their leads and went for our normal routinely walks along the river bank. The mist was just leaving the water, hovering in the warm sun rays; the only sound under foot was my feet treading the undergrowth. My daily routine was up and running, the long night before was nothing but a distant memory, but it could have been so different. Instead of breathing fresh air, with the warm breeze on my face, I could have easily been sitting alone twiddling my fingers, in a stinking pit of a room with closed barred windows, amidst the noise of men and woman crying out.

The water was thrashing away along the river bank, the current fast and flowing, after the torrential downpour from the previous night, so easy I thought to slip over the edge. So easy to fall, and be swept away, how long before the final call, when the curtains are closed, when sleep comes forever?

Dear Shelagh, Beauty my Ugly Rescue Hen

'I am afraid Beauty is not well,' Colin said, 'she has not been moving around, just lying under the hedge. I picked her up and put her in the chicken run on her own with some food and water.' These were not the words I wanted to hear on my return journey from Grimsby after a visit to my parents. I had left my friend Colin in charge of my rescue chickens, and Beauty was my favourite, but it was no surprise to hear that Beauty was not well.

Beauty had slowed down considerably over the past few weeks, her fat body wobbling ungainly up the garden. But, I willed her to keep going, because the fear of losing her was so great, and I just knew the hole she would leave behind would be impossible to fill by another chicken, even though I had been watching my favourite chicken with a huge personality slow down in life, from her zest for living, to now spending more and more time sunbathing in the rays of the warm sun under her favourite apple tree.

I had come to expect this day, and dreaded it with that same fear of loss, and once again experiencing that overwhelming pain that rears up and hits me between the eyes. My heart suddenly felt very sad, a huge emptiness came over me. Tears welled up in my eyes.

I took my suitcase into the house, pulled on my wellington boots, and walked down the garden. I opened the run door, and looked down at my beautiful ex battery chicken that came into my life as a straggly, ugly, tattered; chicken that had been plucked alive, whilst living in a tiny A4 size space, for two of her chicken years. I had four ex battery chickens; three died quite soon on release which is not uncommon because of the level of stress in their living environment. Her beak was and would always remain misshapen, hacked by the farmer to stop the pecking from stress and boredom, but looking at my featherless chickens realised as did others that this practice of chicken mutilation did not work.

But, Beauty had beaten the odds heavily stacked against her; she survived, thriving into an old lady of seven years old. My faithful, funny chicken who walked boldly into the living room, further into the kitchen when given the chance, and further into my heart. She would at every opportunity jump onto my lap, let me pick her up, stroke her, and she has on many occasion shared food from my two dogs bowls.

When I felt stressed myself, or upset, and even fed up with life in general, I would take myself down to the bottom of the garden, and sit on the grass, watching Beauty enjoying her life, sunning herself, dusting herself, chasing the flies, the first to jump on the spade when I dug up worms for her, the first to run after me when I had bits of cheese, or bread in my hand, and always the first to come and lie next to me. The two of us side by side watching the other chickens, watching life, she played a huge part in my life, and now as I bent down and stroked this once proud blossoming chicken, her body felt cold, her head would not move, and her legs given up, sprayed out undignified beneath her beautiful feathered body.

She was old for chicken years, and she would not see this year's sunny warm days, when she and I would enjoy our cheese sandwiches together, watching each other, my respect for her, her ability to put aside those heavy odds against her, and grow into this wonderful creature. I walked slowly indoors, opened the fridge door, and took out a small piece of ham, Beauty's favourite treat, and walked back down the garden, I placed the ham under her beak, she did not move. I knew then that her love, her eagerness, her delight in receiving this treat, had now gone; beauty was on her way out of this world.

It was later that evening when I was lying in bed looking across the fields as dusk turned to night, and night turned to stars shining, flickering in the darkness, as the odd bird or two flew silhouetted against a backdrop of dark trees, also silhouetted against an inky night sky, with the sky behind slipping away to blackness, and as for my mind or my brain activity this went into overdrive once more. I felt an overwhelming sadness slip into my heart, as my thoughts returned to Beauty, alone, cold, her life ebbing away from her, and then my thoughts returned about my row with my sister, arguments with my daughter, and the pain from the loss of my two sons taken from me when they were so young, to be returned as men.

Life was not easy, it was one long struggle up hill, with lots of heavy baggage collected on the way, thrown over one's shoulder, and up the hill more slowly than before, with excess baggage in tow. It's not that we started out in life like this, none of us did, but each and every one of us collects our baggage on our way through life's journey.

My baggage was not always my own making, but other's that I have somehow gathered along for the ride, the ride through life. It was my chicken Beauty, who was now tucked into a bag that is a metaphorically speaking bag, and then tucked onto my shoulder with the other bags. Beauty because she had suffered, I suffered; it was the way for me. And, then I have my sister's baggage, both from Cindy that fills enough for two huge trunk loads, with her life's ups and downs. But, Lisa is something different, where to put her baggage? Well I left it behind, firmly in the lost luggage department, because Lisa was Lisa, a self absorbed, self obsessed Frankenstein Monster created by my parents.

Dear Shelagh, Erik in the Pond

I had my day planned yesterday, all in my head as I walked along the river with the dogs for their early morning walk. My usual routine of feeding animals, cleaning animals, and cleaning my home with my usual obsessive way, and then I would sit down and write up my diary, all my chores were neatly and carefully carved out as I walked back home.

But, just before I reached the railway bridge, my mobile phone rang. It was Helen, 'Mum can you come over here as soon as you can, the puppy has kept both me and Sam awake, and we are shattered. I had earplugs in last night and still I could hear her howling.'

Now I was expecting this phone call sometime, but not quite so soon, not one and half days later. I said I would go over at one o'clock and see what I can do for them both. My visit as grandmother to a pup was sooner than anticipated. I managed to clean and feed my animals, did a little piece of writing, then left at twelve for coffee and toast with my friend Colin.

Unfortunately the cafe or little bistro that is my favourite is now everyone's favourite in St Thomas, a favourite cafe for many, and a long queue formed at the counter. There is no hurry in this bistro, served by one old man, and one Chinese lady at the back, but the food is good, and cheap. I have been known to stand patiently behind the counter waiting and waiting, as the coffee is slowly made, with constant banging from the coffee grinder bashed against the side, to remove old coffee, then the hissing sound of hot steaming milk being made.

We all wait patiently in that queue, no finger tapping's, no feet shuffling, no heavy sighing, no groaning or moaning, just patiently waiting, for the old man to take his time as he lingers over the prices, even though he has done this same job for years, he lingers over the coffee grinder looking thoughtfully at the coffee beans he is about to crush, he lingers over the milk that he gently and ever so slowly pours into the stainless steel pot, then he lingers over the machine, and we all stand ever so still watching this extremely slow process taking place, no clocks, no clocks ticking time has stood still.

But, sometimes I can get lucky and there is no one else standing rigid in the queue, and I can get in first to be served, be it slowly. The food good and cheap, time stood still I walk into the bistro. Two people in front of me, I do a quick calculation with my watch, quick maths on routes, quickest routes to Helens, how fast to eat toast and drink coffee, 'yes it is possible.'

My turn arrives, and I order two lots of toast and two orange juices, because my time has run out to arrive at my daughters for one o'clock. I need to go right now, like last five minutes ago, now I must leave, and orange juice needs only to be poured, and not steamed like hot milk for coffee lattes my favourite and usual drink.

'Surely he can't be slow with the oranges juices, just open the bottle man, just pour out their contents, just go, go, go go, please go, now and pick up that bloody bottle of orange juice, I have to leave,' I think to myself, and then I did what no one else has done ever in that queue, I sighed. Heads turned towards me, the man stopped midway with the bottle of orange juice in his hand, he looked hurt, his hand was not moving, the bottle and the glass had stopped, 'oh my god no, please pour it out, this is my daughter I shall be late for,' I say under my breath, just as the sigh lets go. 'My daughter Helen who herself has to go out at three, and I can't fall out with her, not Helen, because, we are on the road to normal daughter and mother relationship, after years of constantly rowing and falling out.'

My toast eaten with haste, my orange juice drank with fastness that left no taste in my mouth, and Colin still buttering his first piece of toast, I stand up to go, we leave, and on the road to Helen's.

I arrive with two minutes to spare, due to fast driving that had Colin hanging onto the dashboard of the car, and swerving and weaving out of traffic that made a traffic cop look like a novice.

'Oh mum, thank god your here, so pleased you could come, Sam and I are shattered,' Helen said opening the door. I walk into the kitchen, a small, well not so small, bigger than Erik sort of pup sat under the chair. The Northern Inuit, big brown eyes stared up at me. I look around the room, puppy training pads on the floor, no newspaper that I use to have for my dogs. No newspaper, but puppy training pads, like large nappies, with puppy wet wipes, puppy toys of all sorts, puppy blankets sheepskin and woollen. A spoilt pup,' I thought.

'Where is she sleeping?' I asked Helen.

'Well in the kitchen,' she said.

I looked around the large kitchen, 'not good,' I said, 'she needs to be contained in a small space to give her security, like a crate, a puppy crate, then you can sleep while she feels safe and secure.'

After much discussion, and me taking the puppy out to play with Erik and Teigan, I left with my words of advice, 'you need a large crate.' I arrived home a little later when my phone went off, it was Helen. 'I agree with you,' she said, 'but what kind of crate and where from?'

I felt obliged, or rather guilt from the past, but whatever I felt, I agreed to go and buy her and Sam a crate for their pup and take it round later that afternoon, they would reimburse me for it, and surely my act of helping her out would gain me much needed brownie points to get in my daughter's favour.

After more rushing around, animals to feed for tea time, my son to feed for tea time, I left to go and buy the puppy crate from the pet shop. I had twenty minutes to get across the city before the shop shut at six o'clock. I rushed again, my heart racing, my heart pumping, my head hurting, as I weaved and dodged the traffic around rush hour.

I arrived at the shop ten minutes before closing, purchased the large puppy crate, and then rushed over to Helen and Sam's house. 'Oh thanks mum you are a star,' Helen said, and even Sam seemed happy to see me. My brownie points with these two were adding up, to the point where I must now be in credit. I let Teigan and Erik out of the car to play with their pup, which refused to have anything to do with my two dogs, instead hid up under the table, shaking and peeing.

Helen and Sam busied themselves in the kitchen with their large crate, fraught words between them, tension from lack of sleep from this new timid arrival. I sat at their kitchen table and eat pretzels out of an open bag. Helen walked passed me and looked out of the patio doors, 'oh my god,' she yelled, both Sam and I rushed to the doors where Helen was standing, 'what has happened to Erik?' she laughed.

Erik was covered from head to toe in black and green slime, with green slime stuck in his ears; his brown and white coat was green and black, his back legs filthy. 'Looks like he has fallen into the fish pond,' Sam said, bringing a beautiful yellow towel out of the bathroom. I looked at the towel, 'have you got an old one?' I asked.

'No my dad collects towels,' Sam said, and handed it to me, 'we have hundreds of towels.' I tried to clean Erik up as best I could but the smell was overpowering from stagnant slimy water.

I was tired and exhausted when I arrived home, but I had no choice but to bath Erik with baby shampoo trying to eradicate the stench. 'Oh your back,' my son said, as I walked into the house carrying a newly shampooed Erik, 'have you got any freshly squeezed orange juice?' he asked.

Guilt once more overtook me, and I placed a clean Erik in his basket, opened the fridge door and squeezed five fresh oranges for my son, the same time it would have taken for the old man in the bistro to open one small bottle of orange juice.

'You have been busy,' my sister said, when I told her later that evening over the phone what had happened, 'but if their puppy is as timid as you say, then it looks like they have got it from a puppy farm, where it has not been allowed to socialise with any other animals. So sad,' she said, 'just making money that is all the breeder has done. And, with a puppy so timid and afraid, they are going to have a lot of problems with it. Good luck,' she said, 'will you tell them?'

I thought about what my sister said, and agreed with her, both Sam and Helen have had no experience with dogs, and from what I had seen of their puppy, I was inclined to agree with my sister. They have bought a very strong willed dog, a very powerful large dog, which already has problems due its breeding.

'I can't tell her,' I said to my sister, 'they have to find out for themselves, because I know what my daughter is like, strong willed, and head strong, and won't listen to me.' 'Sounds just like their puppy,' my sister said. I expect my phone will ring again soon, just waiting to see what happens next, but as long as I can gain extra brownie points to stay in my daughter's good books then it is all worth it.

The Visit

'The house was different from the other houses in the row, which is why I chose this one to observe. The house had three individual occupants living on three separate floors, and I had to decide which one of those occupants to take, not realizing at the time how difficult this would be. My decision in the end would be the best one for our planet,' I said, gliding towards the lake, a breathtakingly deep blue in the late evening, illuminated by the golden haze on the horizon.

'Go on, I want to hear more about your visit,' a smaller, yet simpler version of myself asked.

'A gentleman of quite some earth years, grey hair, with a heavily lined face, lived in the basement flat, tall, thin; whose nose had a hook like appearance, his fingers were stained yellow from over use of nicotine, constantly rolling up thin, white, paper, sticks that he sucked heavily on, blowing smoke circles into his filthy room. His kitchen window, tiny, position above a rubbish strewn courtyard allowed only slithers of light into his small room, causing him to strain hard with his eyes over his machine. He would spend many an earth day and night, working on his manuscript for his book, his lifeline, his life, and just as dawn broke he would walk quickly to a small shop, returning just as quick whilst constantly looking over his shoulder, he suspected he was being watched, yet it was impossible for him to know that I was watching him. I did not observe anyone else close to him on earth, no family or friend ever came to visit him, yet this was a man who lived in fear, lived on his human nerves,' I said, relishing in my story telling about my travel adventures.

I watched the golden suns disappearing fast over the lake, whilst reflecting on my last visit. I had gained entry into his flat whilst the man had been away on his early morning walk to the shops. I remember how shocked I had felt when I accidently stumbled onto his machine which suddenly lit up flashing all sorts of words at me. It did not take me long to master such a simple device, all devices on earth are simple, but what this man had written about humans did surprise me, so much hate within him. He hated everyone, and everything to do with humans, no wonder he felt he was being watched. His writing was full of murderous thoughts towards his fellow beings.

The man had been some sort of teacher, specialising on how humans live on planet earth, and recently lost his job through age, and this I gathered from my observation of him made him a deeply unhappy human, and very alone. There was one human he did care for, his sister, who had been for many years in some sort of hospital; I found hospital letters amongst his pile of rubbish. He had been trying without success to get his sister released from a hospital for the mentally ill. He was a deeply troubled man, by life, so not my first choice to take, even though he would not be missed by anyone on earth, and my criteria that my choice of human had to be intelligent was met by this man.

I stopped gliding and looked across at the horizon. To my left one of the two moons slid into place throwing pale light over the darkening waters, the other moon behind was slower to appear.

'Why did you not take this intelligent human, who would not be missed,' the small voice asked gliding beside me.

I breathed deeply sucking in our pure air, remembering the filthy chocking atmosphere on earth, 'my time on earth was running out, my decision had to be made soon, and he was so far the most intelligent life form I had come across in such a small area of the planet to observe, and when I made my move to take this man, I stopped suddenly in mid flight when I heard a commotion from the flat above me.

A woman was crying into a small machine she held to her ear, but not for long, the machine was taken by a male and thrown against the window, glass shattered over the rubbish below. The woman ran towards the door, but the male very quickly overpowered her and held her by her throat, her face turned blue similar to ours, but of course for humans not a good colour.

The wonders of our planet never fails me, after time on earth, the second moon was slowly rising; it would not be long before the two were facing each other. The sky would be brighter than daylight, but only for a short time, replacing it with the golden glow from the three suns, between them keeping constant warmth and light on our small planet.

Humans such a strange race, that woman would have died I am sure, if it were not for the man who lived in the flat above the woman. He was a large, bulky, male, the top of his head free from hair which left a shining scalp. His arms were thick, so too was his neck, and ink etched into his skin of varying colours and designs. He broke the door with his heavy body, then half carried half dragged the man to the front door, he threw him down the six concrete steps onto the black, plastic, bags full of rubbish. It was not easy to distinguish rubbish from the man's crumbled body. The male that live above the woman's flat returned to the woman's flat, and lifted her up and placed her on a chair, he fixed the door, and then made their earth tea, the woman became less blue.

A breeze swept through, warm air lifted by the two moons meeting half way in the sky, the water on the lake swelled slightly, no night noises like earth, here it was different, only one species, no need to have the food chain they have on earth, where life forms eat each other, so barbaric, with progress there is no need for this, life here has value unlike on planet earth.

I had been observing this woman through her window, whilst at the same time observing the man in the basement. There was a picture in her room of the violent man that attacked her, he was standing close to this woman, only in the picture he had his arms around the woman's body, she was wearing a long white dress, they were smiling, leaning towards each other. I had not seen anyone else go into her flat and was considering her as a possible choice. She too lived alone, and spent a lot of time at the machine on her desk, the same machine as the man's in the basement below her.

The large man that rescued the woman also had a machine but his machine was bulky and bigger, and all three occupants in their flats, one above each other, would sit at their desks by the window staring at their machines. The woman's desk was covered in pictures of a man she was trying to locate, someone she met when she was very young. She was many earth years old, with long grey hair, tied loosely with red material that matched her lips. The violent man visited not often, and I considered this woman to take; the man in the basement flat left me with some concerns after reading his thoughts on the machine, but the woman was another possibility.

The clearness in our skies with the brightness from our moons means unlike earth we do not have to live by day and night. Unlike earth, time has no meaning here, we have no concept of time, so sad to see a planet's occupants controlled and constrained by its own making of time. Clicking clocks on earth, how they dominant earth life. But, here we are free from such constraints.

Our planet is a small planet half the size of earth, and our life form is very different to humans. We do not have the same physical structures, but we do have the capability of reason and rational, which makes us comparable to human life, and we wanted to get to know our nearest neighbours, planet earth and bring an intelligent life form from earth to our planet, but so far my choices had been two, until that act of kindness from the large man who lived above the woman he helped.

I now had another possibility; he too was alone, although recently he had begun writing letters to newspapers. This man would sit at his desk in front of his machine, observing it with high levels of concentration, whilst holding a piece of newspaper in his left hand, with a picture of a younger version of himself. The younger version of himself held a gun and was dressed in green. The words on the paper were clear, 'Gary Travers missing'.

The paper described the young man in his early twenties who lived with his mother. His mother was waiting for news after his helicopter had been shot down in a war zone two earth months ago. When I took a closer examination of the man's flat whilst he was out, I had a frightening encounter. I had entered the top floor flat, and was startled to find that this large burly man did not live alone.

I caught sight of a brown creature curled up in its own filth, with very little flesh on this species; its bones were sticking out. A long tail move rapidly from side to side when I spoke softly to it, and its large brown eyes with deep sadness within stared up at me.

We glide over towards the water's edge, and the smaller version of myself and I watch my choice of intelligent life form from earth, enjoy the warm waters on its body splashing around.

Of course time was running out and I had to make a decision quickly, my visit to earth near an end. My mission to collect an intelligent life form on earth, one that would not be missed, then impart some of our advance knowledge onto this life form then returning it to earth, in the hope to advance the human race a little further. I had spent considerable earth time studying the three occupants in the building, but all I learnt was how complex this species really was, and asked myself was this race ready for such advance knowledge.

'I like your choice of intelligent life form from earth,' my smaller version of me said, 'it is very friendly. Is this why you chose this one?'

No. It was not my first choice, something unexpected occurred as I was about to take my chosen intelligent life form. It was early evening when planet earth changed from dusk to darkness they call it night. The time had come to make my move and I glide towards the house. But something happened before I could move towards the steps leading into the building.

I caught sight in the shadows a human who I had not seen before walking up the road. I glide to my previous position of observation hidden by our ability to change our appearance to the nearest object, in my case a tree, and observed this human opening the gate and entered the steps towards the building. I watched as this human scrutinized the name plates on the door, then after a few minutes the human chose a door bell and pressed.

The night sky was as crystal clear as the water on the lake, and my chosen one was having a wonderful time on the edge of water, as though never experiencing such wetness on its body. 'Is this the most intelligent life form on earth?' My smaller version of myself asked.

I glide closer to the smaller version of myself, 'oh yes, he is very intelligent. Here throw this for him and he will return it to you,' I said, handing a small round green ball that I removed from earth. 'This creature is called a dog on earth, and he told me he does not wish to return to earth, and not to give the humans any advance knowledge, he believes the species known as animals who live on earth are more intelligent than the humans, apparently the humans are slowly destroying their planet. I have had his food reconstructed for him.'

I watch dog return his ball, his shiny hair covered his body, and his bones did not stick out anymore. Dog bent down and drank the fresh water in the lake.

'Who was the visitor to the flats?' my son asked, as he threw the round green object into the water, waiting for dog to return it.

I cannot be sure who the visitor was, it could have been the sister returning from hospital for the man in the basement, his life would be much improved and not so lonely, if it were her. The visitor could have been the man who had been smiling a lot on the woman's machine in the first floor flat; she would then not need to live in fear of that other man who beat her. I hope it was him from her machine or maybe news for the man on the top floor about his son whether he was still fighting a war or ceased to exist anymore, he was very sad when he read the paper about his missing son, I think he had given up on earth life, and forgotten dog who I removed two earth days earlier.

After the visitor entered the building, I waited a while then heard crying from inside the building, so turned and left. I had some explaining to our elders about my choice from planet earth, but even they felt I had made the right decision. There was only room for one passenger from earth.

Dear Shelagh, A Façade Finally Crumbles

My feet feel alien in their tight black shoes as they touch the gravel driveway; they have been more use to barefoot over hot sands in Malaysia. The car door slams behind me, my last escape route gone. All I can do is follow the driver up large, stone, steps; he knocks on the heavy, wooden, door that shudders around the hollow courtyard. A few minutes later the door drags open, my brother and I are shown inside a dim, icy cold, hallway. We stand opposite a clock that ticks unmercifully loud, its large hands move with slowness, as each tick a reminder of our imprisonment, our lives soon to be controlled by sadistic teachers drawn to the closed world of boarding schools, and where our screams went unheard, our school, a forgotten world to the authorities, a forgotten school.

Footsteps march across the cracked, tile floor, out of the gloominess a figure bores down in front of us. The eyes hold no warmth, a human without humanity, a large woman wearing a white tunic, a face harden from years of institutionalization, quickly removes my brother's small, cold, hand from my own, his crooked glasses too big for his face slip off his nose, he nudges them back into place with his free arm. My eyes follow him, a tiny figure, across the hall, a door slams shut, he is gone.

As the minutes tick by, time without meaning, my turn comes. I feel my eyes well up. I bite my lip; no room for shedding tears, crying is a weakness, bullies sniff out weakness, no time to turn and run. Up two flights of stairs, down a long, shabby, corridor, a door opens her finger points to a bed, 'wait here until supper.' The door closes behind me, shutting my previous life out. I sit on my bed and survey my new world, as silence and loneliness become my new life.

I try to remember my old life back in Malaysia a million miles away, it seem such a long time ago when I said goodbye to my parents. I count nine beds in a row, with just enough space for a small locker. Tomorrow night the beds would be occupied, the official return for everyone back to school. But, for now I have the emptiness, the silence, which is preferable to the room being full, because being full means being bullied again. I was never chosen to be someone's friend, not even chosen to be in someone's gang, or someone's best friend. My sensitivity marks me out as different, oh yes my loneliness is far better than being picked on, laughed at, teased and taunted.

I stand up, walk to the window, tall trees and overgrown shrubs obscure what view might be beyond. I shiver and pull on an extra, harsh, blue, woollen jumper my spare one, now I would be in trouble if I get this one dirty, no change of clothes. My stomach rumbles echoing around the room, it's getting dark. I switch the light on, it flickers into life, a single bulb throwing a pathetic, gloominess around the room, darkening the corners, shadows unwelcome, nothing to do, lost in my own thoughts.

Two sets of footsteps echo around the long, cold, windowless, corridor and down the west wing stairs, the east belongs to the boys section, corporal punishment is dealt out to those that dare take the wrong stairs. A rigorous segregation set in place. My brother is on the east side, he would be eating alone in the cold, draughty, boy's dining room, his little spindly legs unable to reach the hard, cold, flagstones, his small thin frame not unlike my own would barely cover the hard, wooden, chair, no comforts here

The dining room door creaks open; all doors creak here. I sit down in the sparsely furnished dining room, filthy, high, windows, years of rain splattered dirt, allow a glimmer of light to fall on my supper, two single, streaky, rashes of bacon, and tomatoes, one round of white bread covered in margarine, no jam tonight, only the sixth formers got jam, you have to earn your jam, long service and good behaviour gets you your jam, for me it was greasy, tasteless, margarine. I took the piece of bread and lie it on my plate allowing a few seconds before I mop up the juice from the watered down, tinned tomatoes. I carefully slice it up, savouring each piece of soggy bread as I push it around my mouth with my tongue, it would be a long time before food came my way again.

I look across the dining room, on the far table sits my tuck box waiting to be put away, carefully selected by me. Inside the box contains precious items such as chocolate biscuits, and packets of hard boiled sweets. They would not be eaten by me, oh no not for me, they are used as bargaining power, respite from the bullies. The door opens shaking me back from my thoughts, matron appears, two pairs of footsteps up the wooden stairs, down the corridor, and into the dormitory. The door shuts, nothing to do, nothing to see, nothing but my thoughts, my eleven year old thoughts, no one hears you cry. Maybe if I climb under my purple blanket bought in Malaya with my name sewn on, just maybe this might keep me warm, if I have a name then I must be real, because this does not feel real, the sun and the sea back home must have been a dream, best to lose touch with reality, escape is through dreams, to warm sands trickling like gold dust through toes.

I lie awake watching the flimsy, filthy, curtains fluttering across the large gaps from the big old sash windows; black mould around the edges, yellowing once white paint flaking off, so pleased my bed isn't underneath those. I ease my right arm out from underneath the purple blanket, and pull it up a little more around my ears, desperate to prevent the early morning coldness causing me to shiver, have to be careful, must not make a sudden movement, do not want them to know I am awake. The freezing air cuts through my thin nighty, forcing me to draw breathe quickly. 'Is she awake?' a voice from across the other side of the room asks. 'I think so,' a reply responds from the bed next to me. 'Shall we get her?' I hide my head under the blankets and wait. It comes. The blows rain down. I won't cry. The light comes on. 'Time for breakfast,' a prefect shouts, 'get up you lazy lot.' The door slams.

The lino cold on my bare feet, must move quickly to the bathroom, splash cold water onto my face, hair sort of done, teeth clean using pink powder from a round tin, tastes horrible, spit it out, and follow Rose and the others outside the dormitory. We stand in a line holding our black shoes, polished and shined from last night. Matron inspects each pair of shoes, then hands and nails. My turn next as she roughly takes my cold hands and pulls me out of the line.

'Holmes what is this?' she barks, 'black shoe polish under your nails, go back and scrub them, then come and see me after breakfast.' Her white tunic swishes behind her broad back, as she marches away.

I hear the giggles and the whispers, 'you're in for it,' Rose hisses.

Foul smelling soap is useless, against the polish under my nails, made worse by nine pairs of shoes I had to clean last night. The stubborn black refuses to go, I feel the tears well up behind my eyes, the usual taste of salt on my lips. The pain will come shortly, how much depends on matron's mood, 'will it be slipper or cane?' I ask myself.

Every Sunday, rain, wind or snow, we line up in the hall in Sunday best, the nasty woollen jumper on my skin makes me itch, and worse still, it does not block the cold wind, always cold, intense cold, the air is frozen solid, my breath comes out in vapours, like an angry dragon showing off his might. Off we go down the mile long stony drive, walking in pairs, shivering in pairs, the bitterly cold wind chilling to the bone, no fat on me, you have to earn the fat here, the decent food goes to the six formers and the staff.

It's even colder in the church then outside. I see my brother sitting on the back pew, how pale he looks, thinner than ever, and oh no, his eye, above his eye a plaster, the lens in his glasses have been smashed, left eye I think, oh no, can't speak to him can't say anything. Smile, no one is looking, give him a wave across the rows of pews, oh his legs, his thin legs in rough, grey, shorts, they are red raw. He squints at me, his cross eye made worse by his broken glasses, but I think he can see me, wave to him, oh he is waving back, oh no don't tell him off.

Outside, the grimy daylight throws down hail, rice like grains bounce off our faces, no respite on our long walk back, thoughts of steaming, chocolaty, frothy, cocoa keep me focused, as my feet trudge, over, slippery, icy, puddles.

The dining room soon steams up from soaking bodies, ladled out weak tea for juniors; we have not earned the cocoa.

The room is spinning, my head throbs, and all round me heavy silence, deafening, closing in, broken only by my coughing, long and wheezy it makes my chest ache. Nothing to do but stay in bed in solitary confinement, in the sick room, I focus hard across the room, the round bay window, framed by flowered curtains of pinks, and yellow, not frayed, not thin, but lined and heavy. Is that the coach crunching the gravel? It must be Saturday, if I can drag my hot, aching, body out of bed, towards the window, maybe I can see my brother. Footsteps coming, feet feel heavy, chest hurts, need to cough.

The visit not from matron, someone else, someone new, a tall, thin, lady, wearing glasses, thick glasses, she is smiling. 'Hello, my name is Shelagh, the boy's new matron, here drink this, you feel hot. Try to rest; I will visit you when I can, when Matron is away, our secret.' The milk tastes good, she smiles, no one smiles here, I try to smile, my head hurts, must sleep. I hear the coach drive away, all alone, the silence in the room, nothing but silence, the curtains flutter, the draft is cold, my body feels hot the draft feels good, the draft feels cold, my body feels cold, need to cough again

My chest does not hurt as much, getting use to this sickbay with its funny smell, and the flowered wall paper peeling under the bay window, displaying large patches of mould. I stand on the windowsill and look left; I see the boy's playing field, the boy's side of the school. 'What are you doing?' I don't hear the door open, slip off and fall, 'sorry, so sorry,' I say. Not matron's voice, saved, boy's matron, she smiles, 'here are some books for you, and some biscuits.' The door closes. On my bed two books, First Term at Malory Towers, and Five have a Mystery to solve, and biscuits with cream inside. The books feel new, smell new, not a crease in their pages, beautiful books, colourful pictures on the front, the biscuits a whole packet of biscuits for me.

The birds, I hear the birds fill my sickbay full of song, feeling stronger. The curtains dance from warm, spring, breeze, my enclosed world begins to feel a better place.

Dear Shelagh, ARTY FARTY TYPES

My friend Sam who I met through my encounter with the Buddhist center asked if I would like to meet up for a coffee with Sally another one who managed to escape the dangerous cult. Our little trio arranged to meet at the Phoenix at twelve o'clock; as soon as the Phoenix was mentioned as the venue for our little gathering I automatically assumed that it would be a place for arty farty types, with lentils and chickpeas for lunch. I had never been to the Phoenix but had heard of it as Exeter's art center.

I arrived five minutes early, and as usual was the first of our little trio, and wandered into the restaurant area and looked around at the handful of people seated. It soon became certain that I would not be wrong about the menu. The big black chalk board was hung up between the large oval windows; grey December skies threw no light into the room. I had to squint to see the board with spidery writing outlining two options on the menu, spicy lentil soup, and garlic chickpea dip with bread. The tall slim fifty year old woman behind the counter took my order, soup; she was the arts center, with her spiky bright red hair, and numerous rings through her ears, nose and lips, dressed in bohemian style.

I took my seat at a plain brown table and waited, which gave me the chance to look at the other arty farty types seated around me, I could tell they were the lentil brigade, it was their foot wear that gave it away, sandals, in December with brightly coloured socks and loose fitting trousers none descript colour, and these were the two males opposite me, their man bags on the spare seat. Small groups of woman chattered, baggy clothed and colourful contrasting with the December's wet, wild cold weather, I looked up as Sally arrived, years younger than me but haggard looking, her hair unkempt, straggling limp as though it had given up the fight against the gale force winds outside, her pale face was not a happy face, it carried heaps of stress, her eyes seeing everything but nothing, darting around in their sockets like a stringed puppet, the puppeteer gone mad tugging on the strings making large glazed round eyes zip from side to side like a Thunderbird puppet.

She sat down, and was shortly followed by Sam, who at six foot six not fat not thin, carrying a huge rug sack on his back looked like he had also been dragged through a wind tunnel. His hair short and greying fought in opposite directions against each other, his face was red. He thumped his bag on the floor and proceeded to pull out book after book slapping them on the table uttering words that had no meaning only to him.

Sally and I exchanged glances that said, 'do you understand him? No I don't either.' So Sam rambled on, with his manic behaviour with no surprise to either of us, his bipolar disorder worryingly close to out of control, and perhaps another section was eminent. His last book was the bible, he always carried the bible, 'the only book you can believe in,' he said as this too was thumped down on the table.

'I need a coffee,' Sally said, and walked over to the counter to be served by the arty farty fifty year old red haired, Sam followed. I had to stifle my near hysterical laughter as I sat with my friends, Sally who was such a depressive that even she would make the strongest Samaritans hang themselves, and as for Sam he babbled on spilling out words without meaning, random words spilled forth out of his mouth that at times Sally and I talked between us with babbling Sam droning on incoherently opposite us, occasionally holding up one of his books which he would then smack on the table.

My little coffee meeting was taking shape nicely; it reminded me of my time as a social worker, working in the mental hospital with mental patients surrounding me. Sally leaned over to me and whispered, 'so how do you get a personality disorder? Is it nurture or nature?' She was fiddling with her fingers unlocking her hands and locking them, shifting around in her seat her eyes darting around like loose cannons, whilst our male guest jerked forward reaching out for another of his books and held it up in the air, whilst gibberish uttered from his mouth, this man a PHD student, burnt out, his huge brain fried because he was human and unlike a rat not able to cope with the brain's full potential and the power it unlocks when open to all questions about mankind. Poor Sam such a waste, a small window opened for his genius but locked just as quickly now turned to madness.

'Not nurture or nature, but biological and organic,' I replied , 'it's within us all the organic material, and occurs when something so bad happens such as an unnatural human experience that goes beyond any other normal human experience, it can manifests itself into the biological matter that creates personality disorders. My own definition,' I said shifting around in my chair, 'being labelled a nutter opens all sorts of doors for you and is so liberating.'

Sally and I glanced across at Sam who had become increasingly excited when talk turned to mental illness. 'I sit on the board at the hospital,' Sam said, reaching over to pick up one of his books titled, 'The Art of Mediation the path to a stress free life' he held the book up in front of him and read the first page, 'here read this,' he said to Sally pushing the book in front of her. Sally looked at the book her darting eyes made me dizzy watching them zooming from side to side. The book lay open in front of her on the table, no use to Sally.

I glanced around me to see if others had noticed our bizarre little group, our 'nut job' table, but luck would have it, the arty farty types were all busy in each other's conversations, their smooth workless hands making gestures to their fellow guests. My spicy watery lentil soup arrived, served by the arty farty fifty year old, it tasted tasteless no surprise there.

I felt another hysterical laughter rise up as my two friends became engaged in conversation between themselves, a manic depressive desperate to engage in conversation with the manic bipolar who was only listening to himself, and me a personality disorder who lives on her nerves. I concentrated on my watery soup as each spoonful lifted to my mouth but unable to reach my mouth, sliding from the spoon splashing back in the bowl, it was difficult. The two voices next to me raised a pitch higher, each one trying to get the other one to listen, the skies outside were darker as threatening storm clouds threatened to spill cold wet stuff on us bunch of nutters when we returned outside.

Sam was the first to leave, he collected his books that had been scattered across the table, placed them in his ruck sack and threw it over his back, 'I am off, speak soon,' he was gone. Sally turned to face me, her eyes those eyes would they never stay still, 'so do you have a personality disorder?' she asked. Before I could reply Sam had returned, he picked up a book left on the table, held it up, 'nearly missed this one,' he said, and was gone. 'Yes,' I replied.

'Will you get better?' she asked, nervously, because I guess she must think she had a personality disorder given her past, and given her interest in me, and my diagnose.

I mulled over my answer, 'should I soften the blow?' I thought to myself as I looked at Sally as she sat twisting her fingers in a nervous manner, her face, the large black bags under her eyes from lack of sleep, her white frighten face, the nervous energy as she crossed and uncrossed her legs, shuffling in her chair.

'No,' I said, 'you're fucked when you have a personality disorder,' then read horror in her face, and quickly added, 'but it opens doors for you.'

Dear Shelagh, Bid for Freedom

It was time for my little visitor to go, to leave me, and head off into the wilds of the countryside. I felt sad as I fed Spike for the last time later that evening. I put out his usual three packets of chicken and turkey cat food, the best food, he had become of late a very picky eater. In the beginning during his early days of his young life as a baby hedgehog, when he was no bigger than a teacup, I gave him shop bought proper hedgehog food, with wet cat food on a separate dish. And, every morning when I went down to the shed to clean him out he had moved the proper hedgehog dry food to one side, and only eat the wet cat food.

I found him as a tiny baby hedgehog crawling along one hot summer's afternoon, by the edge of the road. I picked him up and placed him in my pocket, I had my two dogs beside me on their leads desperate to get their noses into my pocket to sniff out this funny little bundle of spikes. I could tell he was very young, and was in danger of being run over. I opened the spare rabbit hutch at the bottom in the garden shed, placed some hay and newspaper inside, with a bowl of water and some wet cat food, and left him to recover.

I feared the worse later that evening thinking the shock would have killed him, he was so small, but to my surprise the food had been eaten and he was curled up in a little ball in the corner of the hutch. I spent the following weeks that turned to months to fatten him up and he grew into a fine specimen of a hedgehog, only the cold weather was upon us by now, and he was still not quite big enough to be released into the wild.

I found blankets and old bits of carpets and wrapped his hutch up to protect him from the frosty nights, but still he would come out and eat his food. He was a very clean hedgehog, every morning I would find old bits of newspaper outside his sleeping compartment, only to be replaced by shredded bits of newspaper that he made into a large cocoon. Gradually as the month of November became colder and colder, he made by now only the odd appearance, again eating his food, and cleaning and remaking his bed. Towards the end of December his food remained un-eaten for days, so instead I replaced his favourite wet cat food with proper dried hedgehog food, giving him clean fresh water and making sure his hutch was as snug and warm as I could.

Only on the odd occasion during the winter months did I notice that his food was eaten, but mostly he lay asleep in his huge cocoon that he had made. It was the beginning of March that I noticed that the dry food was being eaten every night instead of the odd week. I began to buy his favourite wet cat food once more, and started the process of feeding him up after his long winter hibernation. I placed both the dry and wet side by side and always only the wet cat food was eaten, and always his bedding was changed every night, old newspaper tufed outside, and fresh shredded and placed inside his sleeping compartment.

March turned to April, and the cold nights were turning to warmer nights, and evidence of hedgehogs visiting my garden appeared. I always place water and a handful of dry food out for the visiting hedgehogs. I would take to going down the garden just before dusk turned to night, and there was my spiky friend sitting waiting by his food bowl inside his rabbit hutch, he showed no fear when I went near to feed him.

The month of April was nearing an end, and I knew that soon my little quiet visitor would have to be released. I wanted to keep him, build a run and hold him where he would be safe, away from traffic, but doing so would also keep him away from other hedgehogs and the meeting of a nice female one. So, with a very heavy heart on the first of May, I went down to the garden for the last time with my Spike's favourite cat food, and removed the long legs of the rabbit hutch and set it on the ground, then I placed his food inside the hutch, but instead of locking the door, I left the it wide open.

I stood at the top of the garden and scanned the semi darkness for any signs of my hedgehog, but nothing moved, there was no sign. Then as the last shades of light vanished leaving blackness, I took my torch to have a look. I peeped into the open shed door, and looked at the untouched cat food and the open hutch door, but nothing moved or stirred in the glow of the torch light, he had gone.

I went back indoors and set about getting ready for bed, and climbed the stairs at ten thirty. I stopped by the landing window and glanced outside, but to my surprise in the glow of the street light, a hedgehog moved with speed along the edge of my driveway, and disappeared into the fields behind.

In the morning, I had hoped to find him asleep in his hutch, safe, but all that was left was half a plate of wet cat food. He had only eaten half and then made a run for it.

I left wet cat food out for Spike in his rabbit hutch for the next two weeks, but he never came back. That was the last I saw of Spike, he has gone, my little quiet visitor who came out at night for his food and to change his bedding was now free to live like wild hedgehogs.

Dear Shelagh, Mystical Village

I would never have thought it possible that I would ever see beauty in a manmade construction in a manmade environment, not me, not someone who found the mountains in Scotland so astonishing they left me in awe and speechless to describe them. Then there is the sea, a constant distant roar of waves thrashing down upon wave after wave. I love sunsets and sun rises with their spectacle of colour, not unlike a firework display as rays of reds splay out across the darkening night time skies, darken misshapen tree shapes on the horizon a backdrop against a gorge of red fire.

So I have never taken much interest in houses, they are a reminder to me of man's vulgarity running roughshod over nature, eating away at green lands to build as the human race multiplies at an alarming rate, with total disregard for animals welfare and their lives. Houses, bricks and mortar to me are a reminder of man's virus on this planet, of what we should not be doing, of what we are about, and how for me this is wrong.

One morning last week, I opened the squeaking Iron Gate to the top of Sherbrook Park, part of it now blocked off due to lack of funding, and the permissive paths granted over twenty years ago to the town's folk of Crediton to enjoy this private estate, is sadly no longer any more. The walk I am about to do before dawn breaks, is on the public footpath route that takes me down the long steep hill about a mile long towards the lower part of the park and the lake.

I went early that morning, not being able to sleep I talked myself into getting up and not wishing to waste the day lying in bed. The time was a little after six thirty, and I could see the dark skies parting way for the rising of the sun, but it had not arrived yet, and only a shadowy blue could be seen. Ahead of me two dogs ran free, I could hear them bounding over broken tree branches, they moved with ease unlike myself with only a cheap torch light for guidance, my feet trod with utmost care. I moved away from the old tall thick oak trees that lined the old path entrance, instead I walked along the grassy bank.

I spent the first few minutes of my walk treading with care certain that at any moment a fall was imminent, then as my eyes adjusted to the darkness, I looked up and ahead, and was instantly transported from the real to the surreal. Twinkling lights danced ahead, rows upon row of them. Crediton town is built on a hill, quite a large hill, and I could make out the dark shapes of houses, flats and rugged buildings, lined with a dazzling display of lights. The lights where they had been placed indicated roads and paths, against a back drop of silhouetted buildings, that now and again twinkled as the occupants within switched a light on or off, as each one started a brand new day.

As I moved closer to the town now straight ahead of me, the lights sparkled and shone brighter, the shapes of trees came into view, just enough light now to make out a tree, but the shapes were many, blacken and distorted, some like gnarled claws poking out from darken corners. Dawn was starting to break and with it a mist rose up from the ground beneath the town, a different picture started to take shape in front of my eyes, like watching a movie in slow motion.

I stopped in my tracks and looked at the mystical enchanted town in front of me, as lights shone out dazzling at times; glittering even, against the back drop of buildings, but with the mist rising up it looked as though the town ahead was floating. There was no breeze, stillness, not even a rustle from my dogs, no sound, no movement; I could have been alone on the edge of this floating town. I was lost in my thoughts, half expecting a white horse to appear with a figure in white and long golden flowing hair, instead another light flashed off and on just a short distance from me.

My footpath, this public footpath would take me in the same direction as the oncoming flashing light, it was unavoidable. Two small shapes ran off towards the light's beam, I followed behind. There were four small shapes now all running around, my dim torch light caught hold of something harsh and yellow, a fluorescent jacket, a shape appeared.

'Good morning,' I said, looking up to a badly dressed early morning dog walker with a torch strapped to his forehead.

'Good morning,' came the reply, 'another one walking a black dog when it is dark,' said the dog walker to me.

'I have a white dog too,' I said, looking at the small brown and white Erik who was being tormented by this owner's black dog.

Greeting said and made we parted company, and I continued with my walk, but the early dawn had now been replaced with grey skies giving off grey light, the town ahead was no longer magical or sparkly instead it was dull drab and overcrowded. I could see a row of lights snaking their way down the hill and towards the main road, worker ants going off to their work. Street light replaced car head lights, office lights replaced house lights, then early morning lights would switch on and the whole process would take place, a continuous cycle of work, eat, sleep and work....and so on... until the time comes when there will be no lights, but a crumbling town eaten away by weeds, and where tree routes push through concrete, when man has long gone, and just the remains of a twisted concrete pole, no light shining now, but through the glimpse of moon rays, black shadowy figures run in out of the crumbling buildings, down patches of tarmac road and into the distance woodland, wildlife in abundance freedom to roam through derelict towns man long gone.

I returned home after my walk, invigorated by the energy I had used along the three mile hike up and down Devon's hills. I had a meeting today, an important meeting, my daughter wanted to meet me for coffee and cake at Dart's Farm, at three pm.

I left the house at two thirty to make sure that I was on time, which I was, well with about ten minutes to spare. I sat at the table near the entrance to the restaurant so I could see when she came. My daughter was on time, accompanied by Rob her husband. I am nervous I am always nervous, afraid to cock things up with my daughter. So, I greet them both with hugs and kisses, we ordered coffee and cake, and we chat, mostly about my daughter's recent holiday to New Zealand with her university friends.

'I have some news,' my daughter said, after taking a long sip from a very over the top hot chocolate complete with sprinkles of chocolate, marshmallows and swirls of cream.

I knew right away what the news was, I just had this feeling.

'I am pregnant,' my daughter said.

I was right, I had guessed, even so, I was still shocked with the confirmation of the news. I am happy for them both, very happy, but also a little afraid, or maybe quite a bit afraid, 'would this be another grandchild, that I am excluded from, not allowed to be near, not allowed to be a grandmother to like my other grandchildren who are strangers to me?' I ask myself.

I hug my daughter, I offer my support, and I am so pleased for her, I just hope that maybe this time one of my children will allow me to enjoy being a grandmother. In my excitement, or perhaps nervousness, I knock my bottle of pear and apple juice over, spilling the contents onto my daughter's skirt. I apologised and wiped away the mess, 'you smash a bottle of champagne on a ship before it sails its maiden voyage. I am sorry the bottle of apple and pear was not champagne to mark the occasion,' I said with jest.

My daughter smiled, Rob laughed, we all smiled, I might have a chance.

Later on that evening I had a text from my daughter, a picture of the scan of her unborn baby, due in May. 'You won't be allowed near your grandchild,' my sister said on the phone later that evening, 'maybe near their dog but definitely not near their baby.'

'Why not?' I asked.

'Because you are a nut job,' my sister said laughing.

My sister's words hit home, and it got me thinking that maybe this is the reason why I do not see my son Carl's children very often, and why I have never seen Alex's baby son, perhaps they think I am a 'nut job,' I think to myself. I sleep uneasy that night, not sure what to expect next year, when their baby is born, more pain and hurt in my life or perhaps a change, maybe some happiness?

BROKEN WORLDS

The clouds broke revealing a patch of blue sky, the first in weeks, or was it months, I lose track of days. I place the ladder against the side of the house, steadying myself against the wind not as fierce as recent weeks; I sit astride the edge of the roof, a pleasant surprise to find no damage. I remove binoculars from my coat pocket, and survey the scene around me, utter devastation lies before my eyes. The patch of sky disappears behind threatening, purple, clouds, a crash of lightening lights up the skies behind me, my ladder jumps, worried it might fall and I would end up stuck on the roof, I leap down the ladder, closing my door just in time as another boom thunders around the valley.

The first thing that hits me as I enter the living room, are waves of warmth cascading through my damp body. I throw another log onto the fire, it crackles and hisses in the large iron grate, sending red flames leaping and dancing into the air, forcing my pot to come rapidly to the boil, smells of lightly spiced beans and lentils flow into my empty stomach.

Before I eat, I have a couple more chores to do. I climb down the concrete steps, and into the cellar, designed like a large spider. The centre houses supplies, various food stuffs such as lentils, beans, rice, tins of fruits, milk long life, almond milk, and soya milk, and many other different items. In ten large sealed containers are spices. Spanning out from here, are four tunnels each one stacked high, with logs, coal, and precious, vital important seeds waiting to be planted, and bags of corn. I scoop out three cups of corn into a bucket, and climb back up the solid, concrete steps into the kitchen area, and make my way to the rear of the long farm house, a large room that used to be a library which now doubles up as the chicken's living quarters. I walk over to the heavy, wooden, shutters and open them, grey light filters onto my beautiful chickens, four golden hens and William my cockerel, they greet me with their usual noisiness. I bend down and stroke William he is unaware, how lucky he is to be alive.

William and my last remaining hen kept hidden when the orders for all birds and fowl to be slaughtered came. The cull, the mass destruction of wild life, left very little in the skies, and what survived soon died off from over anxious people taking careful aim. The air became heavy with silence, nothing fluttered, nothing sang, six months later the rains came. William accepts the corn from my hand, his beak pecking greedily; thanks to him I have an extra three hens to my flock.

I take the broom and begin my daily task, sweeping and clearing the chicken muck. I walk to the back door, unlock heavy shutters, then step outside, remove the galvanised bucket holding water, no shortage of this, and replace their water bowl. I carry the remainder back into the living room, snug from outside winds by my wall to wall books, triple layers in some places, thousands of them, adding extra insulation as well as giving me something to read through long, lonely nights. I remove my lentil stew, then add water to the bowl and place it back on the fire ready for my luxury of the day, a cup of coffee, rationed at one a day, and to keep my day interesting, I vary my coffee drinking times. The smell of coffee instantly floods warm memories of a time living without fear. The bowl still steaming, I place to one side on the large, wooden, heavily, stained oak, desk, whilst waiting for it to cool; I take my reading glasses and search through a pile of notes. My diary of events, my tool to normalization, when normal has long gone, my way of keeping to a routine, forcing my life to have purpose, forcing me to cope with the howling, unrelentless, sounds from outside, when silence indoors bares down like a heavy weight. Thank goodness for the chickens, loneliness made bearable by the company of other living creatures.

'How long has it been?' I ask myself, speaking out aloud, my voice the only human voice I hear. 'I cannot remember,' I murmur to myself; as I pick up the blue diary, flick through pages until I come to the date, August second two thousand and nineteen, and in blue biro the words 'germ warfare spreads east. The attacks have increased, millions have died. Manage to cross the fast flowing ford, driven to the warehouse stocked up on more seeds and corn. Fields turned to lakes. The ford across the road is virtually impassable must buy another vehicle to leave on other side of ford. Have to use the motorboat to cross.' I skip the next few pages, until I come to September twenty fifth, my birthday, and continue to read, 'thank goodness for the boat, it is my only point of access out of the farm. Old jeep on other side doing its job, hired a van and transported more stocks across, not much left in warehouse, supplies unable to get through floods to shops, chaos, panic buying, so pleased I started to do this six months ago.' I went over to the pot and remove the hot water, pouring it carefully onto the coffee grains, then for extra luxury I top with long life cream, allowing the smell to filter through my nose, bringing my senses back to days of normality, when cafes and coffee shops existed, when people chattered freely, before the world became broken.

I scan through pages until I come to December first, two thousand and nineteen, 'electric came on a for a few hours today, listened to radio, bird flu out of control, mass cull to start immediately, all farms to be inspected, all stock slaughtered and burnt, hospitals at breaking point, will have to hide my chickens.' I take a sip of coffee reflecting on that date. I am with clarity able to re-live those horrifying words I heard from my small radio, 'the army have been drafted in, all farms to be inspected, and all poultry to be slaughtered,' my heart race with horror, fear spreads across my body. I remember grabbing my coat and rushing outside, just in time to see an army of jeeps snaking down the hill on the opposite side of the ford. The raging ford would buy me extra time. I rush over to my barn and grab William and the youngest member of my flock Betty; I push them into a box and rush indoors, and down the cellar, shovelling the stacks of wood out of the way until I came to a small opening. On my belly I squeezed through, once inside the hidden back room, I hide the box in the far corner, then squeeze back out, time was running out. I had just kicked the last log back into place against the small entrance, when a voice shouted down the stairs.

I felt my face redden, sweat pouring from me, with slow steps I brushed myself down and walked up the stairs to be greeted by four men dressed in camouflage gear. There was no vet. There was a shortage of vets, instead of gently putting the animals to sleep, they would be strangled or whatever method they chose to use, the quickest taking over any humane form.

'Sign,' here one of the men said, his eyes held no compassion. 'We need to check your premises and your house.'

I nodded and went upstairs, and sat down on my bed, placing my hands on over my ears, trying to shut out the frightened, squawking chickens as they desperately fought for their lives. I don't recall the length of time, and as I read my notes, I did not mention it. All I know was my heart was in my mouth when four men searched through my cellar.

It was later that evening when I crawled on my belly back into the hidden room, and released William and Betty, they must have sensed something, because William who is usually standoffish with his regal display of feathers, allowed me to stroke him, and he eat with unusual gentleness out of my hand.

I take another sip of coffee, and read January first two thousand and twenty, 'the rains have come with vengeance, so too the storms, no electric for two weeks, the skies are always heavy with thunder, tropical rain falls unrelentless, going to make one last dash for supplies tomorrow when the warehouse opens.'

The rain starts to beat against the windows, I hear but not see the rain, the windows are boarded up, with heavy, purpose built shutters. I read on, January second two thousand and twenty 'alarmed at how high the ford has become, more like a torrent of water, took over three hours to drive two miles, roads more like rivers, virtually impassable, no tarmac left on main road, gaping holes, thank goodness for this purpose built jeep, designed for floods, cost a fortune but worth every penny spent on it, otherwise unable to drive through flood waters. Fields are now a swirling mass of angry, brown, waters, lakes instead of grass, houses flooded. Few trees have survived the latest round of battering, by hurricane force winds. A handful of people in the warehouse, I load up with the few remaining stocks, grab the last jar of coffee, two tins of coco, four packets of chocolate, and an exceptional thin newspaper that was to become my last. The angry, bubbling ford is becoming too dangerous to cross. Engine on boat struggled against raging waters. Unload supplies. Satisfied cellar is now completely stocked up, crammed full. Job well done, reward myself with bar of chocolate. Batten down the hatches and wait.'

I rinse my empty cup; walk back into the chicken's quarters, Betty sits on another four eggs, hoping to add to my flock. I am happy to sacrifice the fresh eggs to eat, adding to my flock is more important. William comes over towards me; he crouches down, waits to be picked up. With William under one arm we set off back into the living room. A cosy snug room, shaped like an L, a small kitchen just off the main sitting area. My sofa doubles as my bed, just opposite the fire. It took months of hard work, shifting books around, double lining the walls with special insulation, and with the help of two local builders, we triple bricked the outside walls, I remember it well, they thought me eccentric. The roof was also lined and reinforced with special material designed for the harsh winds of the North Pole.

'Are you expecting an ice age to happen soon?' One of the young builders had asked me. I smiled and said 'no, just exceptional weather coming.' He thought I had not noticed when he raised his eyebrows to his mate and winked, thinking no doubt 'got a right one here,' as the days were warm, barmy and sunny, the calm before the storm.

Living in complete solitude for years, I found it important for my own sanity, to try to keep to a routine, and William has become part of this routine. He sits on the edge of the wooden chair next to me, prunes himself while I take up position at the desk to write in my diary. William my companion, and who I talk to, looks at me with his intelligent eyes, as I pick up a pen, open my blue diary, and start to write, 'April third, two thousand and twenty four. I managed to get up onto the roof this morning, the skies cleared; blue patches of sky, still no sun. All around a sea of water can just make out my neighbour Ben, two miles away, not sure whether he is still alive. I can see two trees over on Denton Hill, at least they have survived, I have four left from the small woodland. No other sign of life. Only a strange land of water, far off hills, little islands like mine, visible, just, through shrouded mist, still the eerie sound of lapping water, that ever threatens to end my home, my life.'

William finishes his pruning, starts to fidget eager to get back to his girls. Not wishing to cause him stress, I open the living room door and he takes himself off down the corridor. He does is usual silly mating dance, with one wing tucked into his side he spins around in a circle. I smile and return to the emptiness of my living room.

I pick up a worn, thread bare yellow duster, and dust, the fire spitting and hissing in the grate, the wind singing outside, the rain splattering on wooden shutters, are reassuring sounds that have grown to be a part of my life over the last four years. I finish dusting, sweep around the fire hearth, and return to the cellar and with my torch for light, I check over my stock, it is reassuringly plentiful.

The afternoon light dims through the slates of the shutters. The rain is just but a trickle, I allow myself the small pleasure in opening the shutters, something I have not done for four years, not since the pounding, frightening rains. Reinforce glass allows only the tiniest of light to filter through, but even so, it is for once a natural light, such a long time I have been without it. I stand by the window; press my face tight up against the pane. My huge barn just across the drive took a battering, but extra money, made it possible to reinforce it to, and thankfully it has managed to hold out against winds of such tremendous speed, that made my knuckles go white as I clung to my chair, fear forcing me to close my eyes, as noises unheard of before bore down on my home, like an angry unseen beast unleashing its power, ready to devour anything in its way.

I grab my outdoor clothes, these too specially designed for the extremes of the North Pole, have served me well. I walk with unusual leisure, the winds have dropped to a more steady gale force speed, perhaps thirty to fifty miles an hour, my body bent forward, I reach the barn, push open the side door, and with my wheelbarrow I can for the first time in weeks, replace the logs in the cellar.

A warm glow in my fire hearth makes such tasks pleasurable. I look in the mirror, my reflection a healthy red glow on my cheeks, instead of the pasty, paleness from so much indoor living. My reward for my hard work is to treat myself to bread, baked in the brick oven; such small pleasures once taken for granted, now become pure and utter indulgence. As I wait for my bread to bake, I pick up a piece of yellowing newspaper, January the second two thousand and twenty, my last piece of news from the outside. I read, the words 'bird flu has cut the world population in half. Millions killed in overpopulated cities, ridden with disease from overflowing sewers unable to cope with flood waters. Rubbish piled high in streets, massive staff shortage due to bird flu.' I knew the words off by heart, but still I read on, unable to digest the coming of the end of the world as I knew it. I turn the page, 'forecast more extreme weather, whole towns slip into the sea. Britain has shrunk further with the sea encroaching inland, flood defence useless. Holland gone, Bristol loses its battle, the sea wins, many die in their beds as coastal erosion eats away at the land. Millions forced to flee to cities; Birmingham at bursting point, instead of death by drowning, death by bird flu awaits them.' The last sentence obviously written in haste, in this flimsy newspaper had so many spelling errors, which still make me chuckle, if only to keep me sane, I smile, and read, 'Armageddooon is here.' Three ooo's instead of one, is the final and last piece of writing on my last newspaper, my last link with the outside world, followed by a small cartoon, of a man on a raft, his white sail with the words 'beam me up Scotty', written in black.

I look up from the newspaper, and realise that night has fallen. There is no dusk or dawn, no seasons. The night's blackness comes at once, as though the outside world has closed, shut down for the night, no warning, daylight is the same no sunrise, no differing colours that nature use to throw in a grand spectacular display of reds, orange, and pinks, instead, blackness, or greyness, nothing in between. I close the shutters; pull the sofa out to make my bed. Collect my duvets, full of light goose feathers, the fire will die down through the night, my bed clothes are warm enough. It's the isolation, the loneliness that bears down like a heavy burden. No time to feel pity, sorry, or sad, instead I pick up a large book, a map of the world, beautiful photographs of world iconic images, mountains, beaches, and birds, so many birds, 'how many left now?' I wonder out loud. My eyes feel heavy, I fall asleep.

A flicker of hope for humanity

A slight burning sensation on my left cheek awakes me. I blink several times before my brain engages as to what might cause the burning through the pinhole gap in the shutter. My senses fully awake, I rush over to the shutters and with fumbling fingers I unlatch them, they swing open, allowing a welcoming flood of sunlight that beams a dazzling array of light into my living room, which picks up dust particles and carries them dancing through tunnel loops of light, a sight so very rare for many years. From the other end of the house, I hear a full bellowing cock-a-doodle-doo, unlike his usual pathetic early morning sound of a cockerel going about the motion without his heart in the job, as though there was no morning to sing about.

I hastily rewrite the list of things to do for today. I always have a list, it keeps me occupied, keeps me focused. Number one, plant grass seeds, corn and wheat, and number two, if still daylight left go to the edge of the drive and check on water levels.

I eat with speed, normally I take my time savouring each morsel as though my last, anxious to make the most of the sun, an extremely rare phenomenon, I rush down the corridor towards the library, and find excited chickens clucking around my ankles for their feed, except William who sits on top of his hen house, pruning his feathers glowing in the rays of sun.

I gather my spade, my trays of seedlings and set about clearing a patch of earth in what use to be a flowered front lawn, but now a soggy, boggy, quagmire of earth. As the sun's rays penetrate my back, I am thankful for the special clothing that protects me from the harsh ultraviolet light. I am optimistic that the sun will very quickly warm the ground, giving hope that the seeds might germinate.

Late in the afternoon, I have no idea of the time, but as the sun begins to dip this alerts me to how much daylight is left. I leave the safety of my sheltered front garden and walk past the barn, and the four remaining oak trees, towards the mile and half long stone drive, which I have watched over four years disappear under water, whilst fearing for my life. I have never felt more alone then I do now, as I proceed to walk against a wind still at gale force, but gentler than previous years, with nervous anticipation as to what I might find.

I had been luckier than most, as a climatologist my passion for weather patterns led me to meeting Ben the same age as me. We had met at university, and together we discovered something extraordinary, a weather pattern that threatened mankind. We had tried with desperation to obtain funding to progress further, but without success. I remember that day so vividly when we had been informed by the department head, that our funding had finally dried up, and without any real job prospects, we sat opposite each other gloomily staring into our empty coffee mugs, whilst the sun beat down through the windows in the noisy student canteen.

'It is difficult to make anyone believe us,' Ben had said, 'I mean, look out there, the sun shines, all seems normal.' I followed his finger as he pointed to the students sitting on the green lawn outside, laughing, reading, drinking, 'where we wrong?' I asked hesitantly, before Ben could answer, my mobile phone rang. The call, that unexpected phone call, was the life line we had dreamed of. An eccentric billionaire, a friend of Ben's father agreed to our research. With unlimited funds at our disposal, we could prove that extreme weather patterns were forming, which would cause great destruction to our planet within six months. But with bird flu rearing its ugly head at the same time, we went ignored, written off as cranks and nutcases.

The billionaire friend did not ignore us, and as a reward for our work, and for alerting him to the dangers to come, the billionaire gave us funds to build our own fortress, so that we might have a chance to survive. We located two isolated farms, two miles apart on a high ridge of the Welsh border. We worked solid for days and nights stocking up our purpose built cellars, reinforcing our homes, and with Ben's contacts were able to purchase clothing and materials used for the North Pole, which would increase our chance of survival.

I had argued with Ben, that we should stay together; I feared the loneliness more than he did. His words still haunt me today, 'we have more chance of survival with separate homes, and stock, then two of us living together and sharing. Be patient and wait it out until I signal you from the roof,' he had said.

I stumble as I step into a hole submerge with water, jogging me back to reality. I stand at the brow of the hill, the edge of the drive; surprise that I am able to walk a few meters further. Four months ago, when I had battled the raging winds, to check the water levels, foaming, angry brown waters lapped at this point, now giant boulders block my view, lifted as though pebbles and carried here by surging, raging, torrents of water. I am aware daylight will be gone, night will fall with instant pitch, blackness, nothing to guide me back, and if I take a wrong turn I could slip into these violent waters and be swiftly carried away by dangerous undercurrents, mini whirlpools that sweep you further into more dangerous larger pools. In the early days, cars, trees, cows swept before my eyes, dragged under, never to resurface. But, I need to look, have to see for myself, whether my efforts of planting this morning were worthwhile.

I struggle up the nearest and largest granite boulder, my feet slip on green slime, I feel something sharp cut into my hand, blood oozes from the wound, with one last pull, I am up. I open my mouth to speak, no words come out, the sight in front of my eyes shocks me into horrified silence, was nothing like I expected to encounter. I am on the edge of a large lake that use to be a farmland below, a valley nestling between the mountains in the background, now all land is covered by one mass of water.

I feel very alone, vulnerable, humble, in such a landscape, my thoughts turn to Ben, 'would it be worth the risk to take the boat to see him?' I ask myself, as I scramble back down the boulder. I argue with myself on the walk back to the house, 'wait for the rains to stop,' he had said, 'for at least a month after they finish.' A month was very long time, when you have only yourself to live with, so tempted to take the boat, the waters look so much calmer. I had hope to see the flag flying, his signal to come over by boat, when I had been on top of the roof, now fearful he might not have survived, I feel I have nothing to cling on to life for, emptiness lies ahead, a vision of nothingness, a world without beginning, a broken world. Who would have thought when the world became broken; the hardest thing would be living with loneliness, coping, with only yourself.

Aware the sun is dipping rapidly, darkness will soon engulf me, like an invisible hand, I ease my pace, besides what have I to hurry for, better to lose myself in the inky waters, better than being alone. I slow down. I sit on the nearest fallen tree, darkness drops out of the sky. I give up. I shiver as the wind picks up and cuts through me, a smattering of rain, falls, mixing with my tears from my eyes, salt enters my mouth. I close my eyes. 'Time to go,' I say aloud, 'time to sleep.' I hear the noise, eerily carried through the wind in the darkness, William's cock-a-doodle-doo. I stand, and follow the sound until I reach the safety of the farm house, and bolt the shutters behind me, shut out the dark, shut out the night.

There is only one thing for it, when I have moments like this and that is to treat myself, and with the light from my torch for guidance, I go in search on the top shelf in the cellar, until finally I locate a jar. Back at my desk I wind my lamp up for power until pale light illuminates the room, throwing familiar shadows into the corners. I open the jar; wait for a few moments to allow the fragrance of heathers to fill my senses, and then gently this gold dust, this honey is spooned with love, and care onto bread, sending memories of moorland, meadows of summer flowers, and bees, summer's warm breeze, birds singing into my living room.

One last thing to do before bed, even though tiredness creeps through my body, I have to write in my diary, have to keep track of days, even though time has gone, records must be kept, especially now, important to keep track of the sun.

Too tired to close the shutters, for the first time in four years I leave them open, if only to hear the patter, the tapping of rain drops as they splatter against the window. Unlike previous thundering, frightening, full pelt of rain over the years, tonight, a gentler more soothing sound lulls me to sleep.

A warm golden, glow, fills my room, waking me from tormented sleep, rays, lots of rays, sun rays; fill my room with warmth, forcing me from my bed, I gather years of unwashed, filthy clothes, fill a bucket, and place over the fire. Whilst waiting for the water to heat, I feed the chickens, and then make a washing line across the front garden using fallen branches to hammer into the ground, with hooks and wire; a makeshift line is ready for my soapy, hot, clean clothes to flutter for the first time in years in the breeze.

The sun still high in a cloud free sky, I remove my clothes, feel warm water on my skin, feel tingly, feel clean, feel free, feel alive, feel hope, washing in the small warm pool behind the barn. Time still left, I busy myself within the twelve foot rectangular wall, reinforced like all the walls, on the south side, all areas untouched by flood waters, utilised to the full, maximise for the full force of the sun. Ben and I knew the direction the winds would come, the wall protection from nature's force to grow seeds, to till the land, to protect the land, to survive off the land. Hard work, I clear and shovel the earth, warm soil between my fingers I plant more seeds of varying kinds, in the far corner, I shovel a patch of earth, and plant snowdrops, tulips, marigolds, sunflowers, and many more, with hope that bees might find their way once again.

With steaming coffee, I sit and watch as chickens enter their new world, they peck, they scratch, they hesitate, unsure of foreign soil between their claws. I savour the last dregs of my coffee, rinse out the cup, then walk over to the barn and sort through various manual equipment, Ben's idea, 'go back to basics' he had said, 'learn to plant, to grow, and mill, but most importantly learn to use manual equipment.'

I roll a heavy green cover back, revealing, a hand grinder to mill wheat and corn to flour. I set about sorting out equipment, a chance of survival made easier by old fashioned technology, no electric needed, no computers, back to basic, back to living off the land, satisfied all was in good order, I walk over to the back of the barn, hidden carefully inside a metal box, a rare piece equipment, solar energy, simple but effective, turning sun into enough power to heat a house, no need for coal, or wood, just sun. 'Sun power,' Ben had said, 'you keep this with you; keep it safe, our future. With food from the land, solar for energy, and us, mankind might just survive.' I remember fighting back my tears, my arms around his neck, his breath on my face, 'only apart will we have more chance,' he had said, 'you take care of the chickens, and equipment, I will take care of our cows'.

Sunlight dwindles, the chickens return inside to roost, I sit on a fold up chair by the door, and allow myself a few minutes of pure simple pleasure, as the watery sun's dying ray's dance over my face. 'Tomorrow another day,' I say to myself, 'tomorrow, or maybe the day after that, or the next, but someday the flag will fly on Ben's roof, and then together at last, time to bring new life on a new earth, for a new beginning.' The sun disappears, darkness falls, and moonlight shines on fresh tilled soil, time to go indoors.

I close the door behind me, but no shutters tonight. 'Goodnight William, and girls,' I call out as I step into their room. I stand quietly by the door not sure at first if I hear correctly, it comes again, now I am sure, the sound, the noise, like music to my ears, my heart skips a beat, it jumps, cheeping, chirping noises come from underneath Betty; she moves, with pride, displays four little chicks to greet a new world.

I pick up my biro, and write, 'April fifth two thousand and twenty four, the sun has appeared for three days in a row between showers, not the continuous downpours of torrential rain like the past four years, but instead, friendly rain, friendly showers with sun. I am not sure if Ben's flag will fly, I can only hope he managed to survive, but I shall go everyday to the roof and look. I am not sure what is left of the world I use to know, but I am certain it will be a very different world to the one four years ago. Hopefully a few like myself have survived, a handful of humans, building a brand new world.'

Broken Worlds

The moon the only light for guidance does little to show the way, my breath is heavy, lingering gasps, the pain in my belly flows through my body as though stabbed by hot, fiery, rods. I want to scream out, but certain death stops me from doing so. I stand at the edge of the wall, crumbling bricks, and masonry litter the ground. Another wave of pain forces me to grip the jagged bars with bare hands until my palms turn red with blood; darkness falls, as gathering clouds hide the way. My foot catches on scattered litter, a wild dog growls in the shadowy corners of the filth ridden courtyard, how much further I cannot remember, time stands still, another growl, a wave of pain, scratching noises from the ground, I let go of the bars, and stumble into the opening, like a wild beast, my long, black hair tumbles about my face out of control, as is my pain, my long brown dress covered in blood.

A wave of unbearable pain shoots through me, I feel myself scream, a hand over my mouth, a pit of falling, blackness, then nothing. Rough blankets underneath my body, do little to stop me shivering, my eyes try with desperation to focus, two faces come into view, friendly faces.

My mother leans over me, 'lie still, not long, don't scream, here bite on this,' she whispers in my ear.

I reach out; grab her hand, squeeze tight; I feel the need to push. I hear another voice, gruff with displeasure; 'she can't stay here,' a male's voice calls out from within the shadowy corners of the water tower.

'She has no choice, they are searching for her. You agreed three days,' my mother's voice, fights back, desperation and fear leaves her breathless, she sighs heavily, then squeeze my hand once again as though trying to reassure me, it does not work, I bite hard on the filthy rag placed in my mouth, a wave of pain, I push the rag away, salty tears fall like streams, mix with saliva enter my lips.

One last push, a high pitch wailing noise slices through the air, a rush of busyness, a few minutes later a small bundle in my arms.

'You have made history,' my mother says, kneeling beside me, her hand gently strokes the small bundle of life. 'Skyline must have made a mistake. I have heard of it happening, but never in my lifetime, you're the first.'

The sound of Skyline forces me to hold my little bundle of life close to me, instinctive protectiveness gushes through me.

'She can't stay her any longer than three days, we did not plan any longer, if she dies so be it, but she has to go after three days. Otherwise she will get us all killed, it is not safe, they will hear about this, they have spies everywhere,' Ulga's voice high pitch with anxiety.

'We agreed the baby stays for three days, but Elena well we did not plan for this, she has lost a lot of blood,' my mother argues, with a force smile, 'the ground troops of Skyline's capital are some distance away, we have a few days, please Ulga let us stay?' my mother unashamedly begs, for our lives depend on Ulga's decision.

'A name,' Ulga says changing the subject, 'it is a girl. She is the first baby born by one of us, it is a miracle, how she manages to produce a baby when all girls and boys are sterilised at birth. She is a real mother, to a real baby, something I have only heard through distant stories, a natural mother not a work mother.'

I feel another tear fall from my eyes, not willing to let go of my baby, I let them slide down my cheeks. The word 'mother', something Skyline's capital had constructed to watch over us when we enter Fieldings, at the age of seven, handed over to woman whose role to guide us into our lives outside Skyline, where we had been produced as workforce on the lands, socialised in harsh conditions through, beatings, fear and hunger. I had briefly caught a glimpse behind Skyline's walls, a place of shiny buildings along clean tracks, horses the only means of transport for the ones in Skyline, for us we had only our legs to walk, our homes created from buildings left over from the aftermath of the third world war, shattered, weed clad concrete shelters, filthy homes, for filthy workforce on the lands.

I open my eyes and hold my baby's tiny hand counting five perfectly formed fingers, I had been lucky in escaping sterilisation. I remember an earth shattering explosion created by an earthquake that sent our escorts scurrying, when we were being taken in large groups to sector nine for sterilization. As the tiniest of the group, I lay flat on my belly and scurried across the gleaming, black floor until I came to a small shaft in the wall, bent over like a small bundle of rags I watched on at the chaos around me, when screams and anxious bodies milled and mixed with children, I had manage to escape sterilization, forgotten in those vital minutes.

Feeling weak from so much blood loss, I close my eyes and listen to the gentle sounds of my baby breathing, smelling her new born baby smell, dripping sounds of water in the cold storage tank cut through the silence. The water tank, this tower had been prepared for my birth date, over the last few months, precious drinking water had been drained and redirected through ancient pipes underground.

The water tank, high up off the ground, an enclosed concrete storage unit had water pumped into it once a month for us Fieldings. We were a close band of people trying to survive in harsh conditions outside Skyline's city walls, artificially selected, we were bred for managing the fields, supplying the food for city dwellers, it had been said, again by stories past down, that our area of twenty miles long by ten miles wide enclosed by a fifty foot wall, was all that stood between us and certain death outside of this, a barren, desolate waste ground, contaminated by nuclear fallout during the third world war a century ago, our world was a broken world. The population ruthlessly controlled both inside and outside the city, because futile land scarce, for crops to grow, limit sustainability of life, and all of us who were entitled to live, bore the mark of a tree on the back of our necks, this our passport to food and water.

My baby snuffles, a hand removes her from me, too tired to fight, my arms go slack, a candle flickers on an upturned iron pot, throws distorted shadows across the round tower, whispered words in the background, my brain too tired to digest, instead I shut my eyes, through jumble thoughts I hear words utter from my lips, that brings about a sudden eerie, horrifying, quietness within the confines of this small space.

'Must go to the wall, got to get out, he is waiting for me,' I say, my secrete out, but my brain, my jumbled brain forces the words like a dam waiting to burst, the words, these life changing words gush forth unstoppable from my mouth, 'I need to go, he is waiting for me.' I try to sit up; large hands push me down a little too roughly.

I feel someone near me, 'my baby,' I call out again, 'where is she?'

'Who is waiting for you?' my mother asks anxiously, 'you know relationships are forbidden punishable by death, no one is waiting for you. It is impossible for you go behind the wall,' she said, louder this time as though stamping her authority, reinforcing her words to Ulga, and the shadowy faces nearby.

I open my eyes; Ulga's face is close to my mine, her eyes hard stare deep into my own. 'She is delirious,' my mother says her voice husky, sounding a little too false, not at all convincing, 'she doesn't know what she is saying.'

'Does she mean to go into Skyline's city wall or outside our wall behind the fields, and into the waste land? Ulga asks, hesitating, 'I mean,' she pauses, sucks in stale air between her lips, lowers her voice, 'no one goes over the wall either into Skyline or into contaminated land, either way you die. And what is this about a relationship? All relationships are punishable by death, not just for those involved but those that know about them, they die too, stunned, then dragged through the streets and left to die a rotting death for all to view. We have all seen this terrible sight, and now we are all putting our lives at risk, but it was agreed, she had the baby kept it for three days, that was all three days, then it must go, we have made arrangements for it, it is too young to feel pain,' Ulga added in a softer voice, 'it was agreed, three days only. Enough time for all of us to experience this new life, although it will be a short life.'

Too weak to fight, I try to sleep, another day tomorrow, three days to get strong, three days to be with my baby, must get strong, must find a way, must leave and find Ram, I drift off to sleep, with thoughts of Ram's strong arms around me.

Through flitted sleep, Ram's face comes into view, his short, blonde hair, a chance meeting, luck or fate, our fate perhaps, certain death if caught, but our love kept all fears at bay. I was different from the other Fieldings, I had a certain curiosity of life, a passion for seeking out answers, looking back I realized that my escape from sterilisation, had awaken me from conditional programming, instead of being brain washed like all the other children by Skyline, our emotions removed, thrashed out of us, gone, taken from us, taught that the weak must die, a small part of me remained alive.

As I worked the fields, I realized my head was not bent forward like the rest, mine was looking around, my fingers poking away at the earth, feeling the soil, feeling alive, and during rare times on my own, I looked around the base of the towering wall that kept us safe from contamination. The other wall, Skyline's wall held no interest for me, I had no wish to explore that wall, but the far wall, the one that surrounds the fields, this was constructed differently, made of lose boulders, sharp misshapen rocks, so different to Skylines smooth symmetrical wall.

On days alone, I would wander to the wall along the field, and touch the boulders, and with my hands outstretched, feel the misshapen rocks, and scrape away at the earth between the boulders. Then as I made small ledges up the wall, I would step up each one, and gradually over time with much scraping, and slipping, I climbed, until my feet were dangling over the other side.

A barren, red landscape lay ahead, it did not look like certain death, so gently, very gently I climbed the other side, and over days and over weeks I explored along the wall, until one bright summer's day, as the dying rays of the sun closed down for the night, I noticed, far off on the horizon, a glowing red formation. As my eyes focused, I notice for the first time an out crop of rocks to the west side.

My secrete safe, I spent the days of summer months venturing further and further west, until I reached the out crop of rocks. My hands now harden, my technique greatly improved in rock climbing, I scaled the boulders with ease. My efforts paid off, I gasp in surprised at the lake below. Water a rare, precious, commodity, rationed in Fieldings used only for drinking, but here was water the size of Fieldings, with trees surrounding the far side. I scramble down the lose boulders and rocks, until I reach brambles and shrubs, not seeing a way through I was about to turn around and go back, when out of the corner of my eye I noticed a small narrow path leading to the edge of the water.

Fear did not enter me as I removed my long brown dress, and bathed in the blue waters that felt strange to my nakedness, we never bathed in waters in Fieldings, my last bath was in Skyline just before leaving the city, no one ever bathed, we had very little water. The water was warm to my skin, it felt tingly. I stretched out on my back, and flapped my hands gently to keep me afloat, and allowed my long hair that fell to my waist to float out behind me, drinking in the beauty around me, drinking in the feeling of cleanliness, feeling alive.

I was lost in my thoughts of pure and utter bliss, and was startled to hear a splash behind me. Two eyes locked into each other, stunned with shock. He was also naked; his broad shoulders above the water, his blonde hair cut short immediately instilled fear into my heart. Only city dwellers had short hair, not Fieldings, but if he was from Skyline then he too faced punishment by death, no one was allowed out behind the city walls, for fear of bringing back contamination to the rest of the population.

He smiled at me, and waved, I dived below the surface, then shot back up, his nakedness below the water confronted my eyes. Red with embarrassment I splutter out a greeting. He swam with ease towards me. Neither of us spoke for a while, each content to enjoy the warm waters, the trees dancing in the breeze, 'if this place is instant death, the let it kill me,' I think to myself, as we swam together along the edge of the lake, silence broken by splashing water as our arms glide through.

I feel my skin tighten, and shiver. 'You go out first,' he said, 'don't worry I won't look, it will be our secrete,' he said, putting his finger onto his lips.

Water trickles on my face, not from the lake, but from my mother who tries to make me drink. 'Wake up,' she says; pushing a container near me, 'your baby is stirring she needs feeding.'

Maternal instinct kicks in, and without any previous knowledge I feed my baby. As she feeds I stroke her small round head, her eyes tight shut, love flows through me towards this small life form, created naturally, not within the Skylines city walls, in giant steel containers, sorting out the weak from the strong, discarded as though junk, then again as children grow up, more weeding out the weak, until a certain standard is reached and allowed to move through to Fielding or Skyline, depending on their test. As I had felt my baby grow inside of me, I began to realise, have thoughts of my own, that perhaps producing humans in tanks, then weeding them out as they grow, was the same as working on the soil in Fielding, only instead of producing a certain kind of crop, Skyline produced a certain kind of human. I heard that it was the only way to make sure human life survived after the third world war.

'Ground troops are closer now, they are searching every building, we must take the baby tonight, it has to go, then she can stay here on her own, and if they find her then so be it, but if not she may have a chance,' Ulga said, shuffling from leg to leg impatiently, standing close to the tower's entrance.

I looked up at Ulga, 'please let us go, let me take my baby, give us a chance to escape, she doesn't have to die?'

Ulga moved closer to me, 'we have no choice she cannot live, besides she has no stamp on her neck, she will stand out as being different, and as you know each of us is counted for, she will never be able to survive in Fieldings, besides it is too risky for all of us. She will die a quick death, no pain, she will sleep for forever.'

Ulga moved back to the entrance and turned her back on me, she bowed her head, her shoulders raised up and down, a sobbing sound, a hand from another Fielding went towards her, she brushed it off, 'this baby has given us something, even in her short life, that none of us has ever experienced before,' my mother said, 'we are learning to love another human,' my mother sighed and leant over to touch my baby's cheeks

'It is called compassion,' Ulga said, 'I have heard of this, but never knew what it was until now, until this birth. I too feel so sad but she has to leave us, or we will all die, and then compassion will not be passed down.'

My baby finished feeding, I lay back and hold her close to my chest listening to her breathing; pain wells up in me, knowing that she will never experience the lake, the trees, and the freedom of life that I had experienced not long ago, where she was conceived.

Ram and I met often down the lake. I was always first in the water, and he would swim over to me, neither of us speaking of our lives inside the wall. He would always wait until I left the edge of the lake and walk back up the rocks before he dressed. Strangely I never saw him wearing clothes, he was always naked. It was only towards our last meeting, when my stomach had started to swell, that I had noticed something red tucked away out of sight behind a shrub, it was only by chance that I caught sight of it, just as a small furry creature shot up a tree, and then my eye saw the red garment on the ground. I felt faint with fear and clung onto a branch, a few minutes later I dressed and returned to the wall.

On my way over the wall back to Fieldings I could not bring myself to think about his red tunic, surely a mistake, I must have been mistaken, only ground troops wore red tunics with black trousers, and black helmets, they had the orange tree of fire emblazed on their backs, the tree of fire was instant death to Fieldings, usually it meant punishment when they entered our homes. We never saw their faces, black full face helmets kept them hidden, but they would from time to time ride through our area, search our broken down buildings, then drag out a helpless Fieldings and in full view of everyone, stun them, then leave them to die a slow lingering death as a reminder of what would happen to us, if we should step out of line. We never understood the nature of the poor victim's crime, it was not for us to ask any questions; instead we would lower our heads, feel relief that this time it was not one of us.

Ground troops always rode on horses in groups of fours, and always when they arrived, someone would die, and now they were closing in searching for something, which was unusual, normally they would ride straight to their killing. 'Why are they searching?' my mother asks, a question we were all wondering about, but to afraid to voice openly. 'They would not know about this birth, and certainly I have never in my life heard of them searching, this is most worrying,' she said sighing, her sweated brow knitted together, she rubbed her hands on her brown dress, filthy like my own.

'We have a short time before daylight has gone, then we will take the baby,' a male's voice said stepping from the shadows, 'say goodbye, to her,' he said softly to me, the gruffness of his earlier voice gone.

I hold her close, tremble with fear and love for my baby; it had not meant to be like this. The morning I was suppose to have left Fieldings for the last time, hell had broken out. I was as usual positioned near the far end of the wall, twenty feet from my climbing point, and ready at any moment to go over. I had been struggling to hide my growing stomach, but the baggy brown dress that we all wore, every dress the same size, the same colour did much to help disguise my condition, and like the rest of Fieldings, I went to work in the fields, the same routine that all Fieldings have, only for me and my baby this would be the last time.

That morning as I bent over waiting for my chance to escape, it proved more difficult than normal, it was an exceptionally hot day, and without any warning I felt myself topple over face first into the field. I do not remember how long I lay there on the hard ground amongst the crop, but as my eyes came back into focus, it was Ulga's face that came into view, lined with fear and horror, it was then my condition became known. A small group of people half carried me to my home, and lay me down on a pile of straw, my bed. Hushed voices bubbled around me, concern etched on grubby faces.

'If the ground troops think she is weak she will be stunned and left to die,' Ulga said, then turned to me, 'you must not show your weakness you must act strong until you give birth.' After that day I was constantly watched by the other Fieldings, someone was always with me, a natural birth was something that never happened, and suddenly I was a 'show piece', normal routine interrupted. Leaving Fieldings was impossible now, my only chance was to give birth and leave quickly with my baby, over the wall, and live alone on the outside. After my last meeting with Ram when I spotted his red tunic, I knew then we had no chance to be together, he had been conditioned like I had at an early age, only instead of training to working on the fields like myself, he had been schooled in the art of stunning, and killing, he had been conditioned to enjoy his work, like I was suppose to enjoy my work on the land.

A rush of cool air returns my thoughts to the present, the tower door opens, a woman rushes in, and her voice pitched high in heated excitement.

'They are very close. Two buildings along, time to take the baby,' the woman said lunging forward, to take my baby.

I hold my baby close to me, and wrap the filthy rag around her tiny body, and like a small doll she opens her tiny mouth and yawns.

'No,' I scream into the semi darkness. Anxious faces gather around me.

'She will die stunned first. You must hand her over, at least we will give her a decent death,' Ulga said, 'no time to argue, say your goodbyes, now.'

I lean over and kiss my baby's forehead, 'leave us, please,' I beg, tears rolling down my face. Ulga reach down and attempted to pull my baby from me, I held on tight with inner strength, the air shattered by my baby's cry.

Her cry, echoes around the water tower, bounce off the watery walls, bodies once stationary, jump into feverish action. 'That cry, the ground troops will be alerted to us, quick no time, must go, leave now,' my mother calls from the door. Bodies push roughly past me, tripping, falling, fear driving them on, until there was only silence, as my baby's hungry cry is calmed by my breast.

All alone, I can only wait; my fear has gone, without my baby there is no point to life, this world, this place, Skyline's city and Fielding's workers, not safe for a new life to join. I listen to the sounds of water trickling through the pipes, soon the place will be flooded with the rationed water, or soon the ground troops will be here with stun guns then lingering death. If I am lucky the water will come first, my baby and I together, a mother's love, a mother's arms will cradle her until such time. My feet feel wet, the water trickles down the pipes, a gurgling, flowing sound of precious water, giver of life, the tree of life, our tree stamped with heated iron on our necks, our right to life, will end for me with water.

I close my eyes and wait for whichever comes first, ground troops or water, my baby suckles contentedly, no idea of what is to come. My legs feel heavy, water flowing fast, footsteps outside, shouts, I hear shouts, a bang, a piecing scream, then silence, until it happens again, and again, three bangs, three screams, the air outside grim with death, the ground troopers must have found them, three shots, three deaths, mother, Ulga, and the man. I hear footsteps towards the tower, then someone close on the other side, the door opens, the red tunic, the black helmet, the fiery, red tree that glistens from semi light from outside. I close my eyes, hold her tight, and wait, it will come soon.

'Be quiet, hang on tight, we do not have much time, others will be here soon,' the ground trooper says, his fingers brush my hair. He scoops me up, I cling to him, my baby tight around my chest wrapped by the long filthy rag. My brain too tired, too exhausted, numb with fright I feel his strong arms around my waist, together we ride through the rubble that was my home, past three bodies, three dead ground troops.

No one will come out of their homes to see us, fear makes them hide away, so we ride past the ruins, past the filth, and on and on we ride, until the wall looms down in semi light.

He gently lowers me to the edge of the wall, then kneels down beside me and whispers through his black helmet, 'wait here,' he says, 'trust me, you must trust me, I shall be back for you, but first give me your baby, I will take her to safety, then return for you.'

I slowly unwrap the filthy rag that ties my baby to my chest and hand her over, 'take care of her,' I say, 'she only has you now to watch over her.'

I watch him climb the wall with ease and then darkness falls, as the sun slides behind it for the night. An eerie quietness descends across the fields, too numb to cry for my baby, too weak to stand, I lean against the wall and watch the stars come out in the darken night. The moon glides behind the clouds, time without meaning when you lose the one you love.

I close my eyes and prepare to sleep, 'he has been too long, he won't be back for me,' I whisper into the night, 'he doesn't need me, he has his child now.'

'Be quiet,' the voice in the darkness calls, movement down the wall. A shadowy figure in a red tunic, black trousers, but with no helmet, 'our baby is safe, come, your turn now, she wants her mother. I will help you over, and then we will be free to live a different life,' Ram says breathless.

With inner strength I climb the wall, and with help from Ram I sit astride the top, 'say goodbye to your old life,' Ram says, as he sits next to me, his strong arms around my waist, 'with your skills working the land, and mine in strength we have a chance, to live outside.'

Ram carries me with ease across the barren land. I slip and slide across the boulders, then as dawn makes its way across the skies; we walk hand in hand towards the lake, then down the small path, past high reeds and shrubs, until we come to a small clearing. I gasp in shock, my hand covers my mouth, I stand and stare, as Ram proudly points to our new home, a wooden hut, nestled between tall trees. I open the wooden door and there inside on soft clean blankets I find our baby fast asleep.

'I have spent weeks, smuggling all this from Skyline,' Ram said, 'we have pots, pans, blankets, and look,' he said proudly holding up the most beautiful fabrics of gold, blue and green, 'we can survive,' he bends down to lift his child, our child, and cradling her close, he says with love 'a new life, a new beginning.'

Dear Shelagh, Four Felt Tips and a Notebook

Two years ago my GP who has been very supportive towards my mental health condition arranged for me to try Art Therapy that had just started up in Exeter. I said I would like to try it, so my name was put down via a referral from my doctor. A week ago, I had a letter inviting me to attend an interview at the Arts Therapy center, this is two years later.

I have to admit I was quite looking forward to it. I had tried Art Therapy sometime ago when Carl was a baby and I was in Salisbury mental hospital for what I now know as Post Natal Depression only then it was not recognised, and I was admitted with depression. It was in the good old days when mental health services had money, and treatment was available, unlike today where only pills and potions are given out by those in the mental health services to dope up mental health patients, it saves on expensive time consuming treatments, and cuts down on the number of staff and hospitals, and therefore mental health patients can be treated in the community, or otherwise known as 'Care in the Community', only we realize, that is us mental health patients, or as my sister calls us 'nutters', no care exists, just pills. And, instead of having a lot of health care officials to take care of your mental health needs, with pills you only need one or two health care workers to dish out the pills, and the big drug companies can then make big bucks. This I learned when I worked in the mental health environment, as a social worker. I have been both in the system as a patient, and in the system as a social worker in mental health.

So, I was pleasantly surprised and pleasantly pleased that at last I had a chance of trying out some Art Therapy, which to me sounded like a pleasant experience, that is to bring out your inner and darker thoughts not with words but through paint, expression on canvas, releasing your demons, and allowing yourself at least to be able to be free to create. At last in my traumatic life I can for the first time actually look forward to something.

Two days before my appointment, I had a phone call from the Arts Center, telling me that my interview had to be postponed because the arts therapist was off sick. I rescheduled my appointment for the following week, and was asked politely if I could go a few minutes early to fill in a form, to which I replied 'yes'.

On the day of my interview for my Art Therapy, I left my house at nine thirty on Friday the 13th of September, to drive the short distance to the arts center, where I was sure to arrive in plenty of time to fill in the questioner. At ten to ten, with ten minutes to spare to my appointment, I turned into the drive of a large Victorian Mansion, which apparently used to belong to the Mayor of Exeter a wealthy landowner. The driveway was long and curved through a wooden secluded setting of green shrubs and old trees, and lawns trimmed with exotic borders of flowers. The house had an impressive entrance with large stoned steps leading to grand double high ceiling wooden doors with a large old fashion heavy door knocker.

I rang the tacky modern bell next to the bronze door knocker, and waited. Some minutes went past when I tried again, a little while later I heard footsteps approaching, whose footsteps they belonged to, were not at all in a hurry. The door was unbolted and unlocked and it swung open, and half hidden behind them, a tall thin man peered at me through spectacles. 'Yes,' he asked. I explained I had an appointment and showed him my crumbled wet paper with my name and appointment time on it. It had got wet because by now the rain had started to fall heavy and fast.

He said nothing more but opened the door a little wider, and ushered me into a grandiose entrance with exceptional high ceiling with a sweeping staircase to the left. The place had various ceramic pots on show, and decorated with colourful tapestry and various art pieces. I followed the man into a large room, and was told to wait. His footsteps retreated, a door in the distance closed and then an empty silence descended into the cold room. Even though the room was tastefully furnished, two brown sofas frayed and over used covered most of the stained brown carpet, the cushions were brown and white flowered. Between me and the high fireplace tiled also in brown tiles, old fashion type with some sort of pale cream decorative flower along the fire surround, and opposite this was a large brown, heavy, wooden table, piled high with books, big books, oversize hard back books that made holding them up to read quite hard work, they were books on the world, wonders of the world, outdoor type books filled with beautiful pictures of awesome deserts, skies, rivers, seas, and waterfalls. And, most interestingly as I flicked through the first book that covered all of my lap and hung over the sides of my legs, I looked at amazement of Iguana falls in South America, when only a few days ago, Chris had sent me a photo of him posing by this magnificent water fall clinging with sheer terror etched over his face onto the rails as the water cascaded behind him.

I flicked through more pages, and listened for any sounds that might come, but there was nothing, just silence. I noticed then that the windows were bolted, and my stomach twisted a little as I looked on at the modern fittings attached to the old fashioned sash window, my thoughts returned to the heavy bolted door, there were no escaping, and still no sound. It was eerily quiet, too quiet.

In the stillness of the large building, my Imagination ran riot thinking through all the worse possible scenarios. Here I was sitting alone in a locked building, and one I had walked into willingly. The only person I had seen had disappeared leaving me alone with a coffee table piled high with someone's books. My bladder already full when leaving my house was now protesting about its fullness and clearly wanted empting. I stood up and walked to the half open door, pushed it further open and looked out into the empty long corridor with doors leading off from it, all closed.

The room I had been shown into was situated in the middle of the corridor, and found myself with a choice. I could take the left or the right, but I chose the left, and located the toilet immediately. It had 'toilet' written on the door.

I returned to the empty room, but on my return was confronted by the man who let me into the building. 'Sorry but I have tried ringing Malcolm and tried texting him to let him know you have arrived, but he has not got back to me yet,' the man said, without any emotion. I looked at the clock in the hall, ten twenty five; I had been here nearly three quarters of an hour.

The man left as silently as he had appeared like some sort of ghostly apparition in this old lonely house. I returned to the chilly waiting room and turned my attention to the outside window. I could see tall conifers out of control, their height towering over the large Victorian building held back daylight, only shades of grey filtered through onto the small patch of lawn, where two sparrows jostled for worms, the rain now falling fast and furious hitting the ground so hard that drops splashed upwards waking the worms. I allowed myself to daydream about nothing, a blank mind, only the two birds kept me from falling asleep.

I was still in this trance like state when I turned towards footsteps rushing towards the waiting room. The door was suddenly pushed open and in tumbled a sort of stick like figure into the room; it only took me a few seconds to read this little man's body language. He jostled and hopped about, totally exasperated, he was clearly rushing, and as he made hurried introductions, I found myself also hurried out of the waiting room and up the spiral sweeping stairs, and hurried down a long, narrow, dimly, lit, corridor and hurried into some sort of art room. It felt as cold and bleak as the rest of the house, even shades of colour on various pieces of paper that hung on the walls did little to lighten or jolly my mood or the room.

The little man made a sort of smile one of those false smiles that mean nothing, but in doing so displayed two missing front teeth. 'Take a seat,' he said gesturing to the large table that dominated the room with hard back old fashioned seats clustered around it, he tried to be discreet but was unable be so, when he searched around the room for the door stop to prop the door wide open. From my own social work training, I knew that safety meant keeping the mental health patients at arm's length and to make sure I stayed closest to the door. To make it easier for him to feel safe, I walked to the back of the room and took a seat leaving the large table exposed between us, whilst exposing this mental health's worker's tactic bare, he as I knew he had no choice but to sit near the door.

With me at one end of the table the far end, and he nearest to the door, the large distance between the two of us was blaringly obvious, too obvious, and then we sort of looked at each other over the stained wooden table from one end of the room to the other. I allowed him to speak first, to which he said, 'I am sorry I am late, but I was told you cancelled.' His words echoed around the large room, I replied 'no I did not cancel, 'I am here.' He twisted around like a hot potato on a spit, he was pushed for time, this was obvious, and he was stressed, his body language told me so, his hands were all over the place, his fingers picking up pencils, shuffling pieces of paper, and he could not sit still.

I on the other hand, sat with my arms by my side, and perfectly still, a deliberate ploy on my part; I had the outward presence of calm. I knew from my own professional training not to fold my arms, or cross them, because in doing so can indicate to the observer that I am not comfortable, so instead I held the relax arm position, and smiled at him. To an outsider it would appear that I was the professional and he my client, and not the other way around.

'Could you please fill this in,' he said sliding a piece of paper towards me. It was the customary questioner on how I feel. I read the questions and ticked the box, self harming, yes, dark thoughts, yes, suicidal thoughts, yes, not able to sleep, yes, disturbed sleep patterns, yes, disturbed dreams, yes, and so on. By the end, I was by this questioner, evaluated as a suicidal and dangerous nutter, and with the ongoing problems with my daughter, not allowing me to have anything to do with my granddaughter; I felt all those things and more. But, I contradicted this with my posture displaying outward calmness, yet inwardly I was a mess of emotions, and sick in my stomach with nerves.

I slid the paper back to him, he picked it up and scanned down the list of questions, and through my answers, until there was a slight smile on his face, on the question as to whether or not I am violent, I had put 'no'. 'So pleased you're not violent', he said, and placed the paper on the desk, in front of him, and then he shifted toward the door and closed it with his foot, then leaned his head on his hands and looked at me. I looked straight back making eye contact, not shifting my gaze. I waited for his next question and I had the answer ready for him. His question soon came, the standard question that all mental health workers are trained to ask, and 'what do you think art therapy can do for you?' he asked. I was right; this was always the next question in any sort of therapy.

'Well I don't expect art to make me better,' I replied, 'but perhaps with my lifetime of pain, it might just give me a moment of peace as I paint, like a small window in my life of not thinking of my past or my future, but being in the here and now,' I replied. His next question was another I was expecting, 'what brings you here?' he asked. This was a difficult question and I fumbled around trying to sum up my life, but this was harder than I thought it would be. As I tried to explain my life to this little man, he rudely jumped in or waded into my explanation, 'please keep it to the point, and don't go off track, 'he said, 'there is no time, we only have an hour.' Each time I tried to explain about my life, he gave me little chance to explain and kept shouting at me, 'we don't have much time keep to the point,' he shouted exasperated.

This little man was clearly in my own professional experience and training as a social worker in mental health, not at all acting like a professional counsellor; instead he was acting on his own emotions, that being stressed himself, and wishing to be somewhere else. Or perhaps he himself should be doing art therapy.

I was getting annoyed with him for continually interrupting me, so much so that I eventually snapped and said calmly, 'I really don't envy your job. I mean us humans are such complex beings, and given my traumatic past, and how this left me a damage person, and you only have an hour to make an opinion of me, must be quite a tough job for you to do,' I said perhaps a little to sardonically, and much to the surprise of this little man, who never expected that sort of response.

He stared open mouthed at me, closing and shutting it like a gold fish, eventually he said, 'well let me explain about the set up is here. We don't have a lot of funding so I have to make sure the people who get the support they need through art are the right people, and you're not.' It was my turn to stare open mouthed at him. 'Time up,' he said suddenly, 'but before you go let me give you something,' and with this he jumped up quickly from his chair and rushed outside, a few minutes later he returned breathless to the room, and handing me four felt tip pens, blue, green, yellow and red, with a notebook. 'Here take these,' he said, 'and do some art work in this book.'

I found myself on the step of the front door, with it closing firmly behind me. I drove down the sweeping drive and out of the gate, and went and on my way to meet up with John for lunch, he had been waiting for me since eleven. I had only expected to be an hour, and if my appointment had been kept to the right time, then I would have made my lunch date with John. I found John sat at the table with an empty large cup, the remnants of a coffee latté showing around the edge of his mug.

'Well how did it go?' he asked excitedly. John knew how much this art session had meant to me, I had been going on about it for weeks. I dug into my bag and removed the four felt tip pens and the small notebook. 'This is it,' I said placing the items on the table in front of him. I looked at Johns puzzled face, he said nothing. 'This is my art therapy, four felt tip pens and this book. This is what I have been waiting for, these last eighteen months, and at least three referrals from my doctor, for these,' I said pointing to the miserable felt tip pens, one had already started to leak, it was the blue one. 'Lunch,' John asked.

When I arrived home I found my neighbour with her small child outside in her garden, I called her over and handed her the four felt tip pens and my notebook, for her little girl. 'Thank you,' my neighbour said smiling.

So art therapy has changed since my days in Salisbury mental hospital. No more painting in a safe environment with a choice of oils, water paints, or crayons, no more weaving baskets, giving us mental health patients a chance to do something creative without any pressure, a chance to relax from our illness, and a chance to express ourselves amongst others who have similar conditions, and a chance for a small bit of respite. It's all gone, the art therapy centre, all that is left is a huge house, an expensive drain on very limited resources, it keeps the two men who run the center in a lavished office, and without the mental health patients the center is eerily quiet, hidden away, with its big box of felt tip pens, and a stack of notebooks. That little man knew nothing about me, if he had let me speak, he would have learnt that I already have a little notebook in which I write my thoughts, write poetry, and try to find some way without heavy medication to keep safe. All I asked was an hour a week in a safe environment to express myself through paint, a soft tonic, soft medication, a little bit of support. Instead, as I suspected, there is nothing out there for mental health patients.

Postscript

Perhaps this should be in the beginning but then it would be a normal book, written by a normal person, only I do not feel normal. I suffer from borderline personality disorder, caused by my early life at boarding school, volume one in my series of Stumbling through Life. I have written my books in the hope that my children may one day read them and perhaps learn to understand their mother. Mental illness is not an easy illness to live with; it is often hidden from others, therefore a lonely illness to deal with. Only it is the family members who suffer too, not sure how to deal with someone who is not termed 'normal.

My writing is often raw and emotional; it helps me to deal with life's problems that are constantly thrown up. My letters Dear Shelagh are letters actually written to a very good friend of mine who use to be a matron at my boarding school. She has been a constant support in my life. My short stories and dressing gown poem are based on actual events that happened to me, but I have embellished them to create a story that goes through my own mind when I am out walking with my two dogs.